The Women's Ward

By Ruth Carter

'One million people commit suicide every year'
The World Health Organization

Ruth Carter

Published by
Chipmunkapublishing
PO Box 6872
Brentwood
Essex CM13 1ZT
United Kingdom

http://www.chipmunkapublishing.com

Edited by Lucy Dow and Mary Dow

The Women's Ward

Chapter 1

Her husband dumped the case and left her at the door.

She wasn't quite sure where she was, only that there had been a telephone call and her husband had driven her there. There was a metal square at the side with buttons and numbers on each one. She peered through the windows in the door; there seemed to be people wandering about. She had nowhere to go, it was too far to walk home and she had no money for a bus with her. She saw a bell on the other side of the doorway and pressed it.

Someone unlocked the door.

"Hi, I'm Sean, and what's your name?"

"R", she replied.

He picked up her case.

"Come on, follow me R and I'll take you to your room."

There was a thin corridor with an array of posters stuck haphazardly to the peeling yellow walls.

It was only when she was ushered into the room that she noticed there were four beds with curtains round them and lockers. She realised it must be a hospital.

"Why did Dave leave me here? I'm not ill?"

"No," Sean replied, "you just need a rest."

3

"I can sleep in my own bed, thank you very much. Let me go home. "

Sean talked quietly and tried to explain that it was not a realistic option.

"It's getting late. Why not just stay tonight and we can talk tomorrow?"

R began to calm a little.

Later he began to explain the procedures for new admissions.

"Sorry but your bags need to be searched in case there is anything which could be harmful. I've brought you a pamphlet which explains hospital rules. There are patients here who try to harm themselves so we need to protect them."

R's brain was too muddled to understand just what type of hospital she had been admitted to and agreed to his suggestion because she needed to sleep.

Sean emptied R's handbag onto the bed. She was embarrassed by the sticky hairy sweets that the children had given her. He took a pair of eyebrow tweezers, a biro and a box of matches.

"I need my pen, I need to write. You can't hurt yourself with one."

"Actually you can. Last month a girl pushed one through her ear drum and punctured her brain, that's why we've introduced the rule."

"Well I wouldn't do that."

"You might not, but we have to be careful."

Sean picked up the offending items.

"Probably see you later; I'm on until ten, then at eight in the morning. No peace for the wicked."

The Women's Ward

He winked at her as he left.

The letters wriggled, the words seemed to laugh at her. She didn't understand most of it but managed the visiting times. She rang her husband on the mobile to tell him that they were seven until nine. She unpacked, and then walked into a corridor.

"Can I have that?" a nurse asked as she saw the mobile R was using to try to explain the situation to her husband. He had hung up.

"Suppose so."

Another nurse spoke to her. R knew her name from the plasticized label pinned to her lapel. It was Sarah.

"I expect to see you in the lounge. You need to socialise."

When R entered the room there was a fat woman in a nylon night dress who was muttering incoherently, "Uncomfortable, uncomfortable."

She was touching herself, her crotch and arm pits, standing in the centre of the room blocking the television from the assistants. On top of her nightie she wore a thick, slightly soiled, woollen jumper, stained with the remnants of an earlier meal which R assumed to have been breakfast, because there were glutinous thick yellow marks on the left side.

There was a girl in black clothes and purple nail-varnish. Another woman spat on the floor. There was a strong smell of milky coffee and toast, with a suspicion of urine.

She looked round the room. There was a fat television which was bolted to the floor and a collage on the wall from a previous Christmas, all torn tissue and deflated balloons wrinkled with age.

A woman stood up and started to shout.

"You bastard, it's your entire fault, you pushed me down the stairs, you didn't care. I lost our baby, and your sister is no better, she's a real whore."

A nurse walked towards her.

"Come on back to your room, can't have you upsetting other people."

It was too late for R; she needed somewhere to hide, the noise and the bizarre behaviour of the other people disturbed her. She found bathrooms and toilets but the floors were too cold to curl up on. What she wanted to do was hug herself away from everything.

She found a room with a flipchart. She hid behind it. All was quiet. She thought she was in hospital but didn't know why, she was confused and scared, too much confusion, she had enough of her own problems. She looked round the empty room she had found. There was an exercise bike, covered with bubble wrap; she noticed four mats encased in a shiny plastic.

She tried to settle down, block out the world around her. She knew now where she might be and was frightened. It was a place where mad people were sent. It would be alright, Dave would take her home after visiting time. The doctors would realise that they had made a mistake. The door squeaked; Sean the nurse smiled at her.

The Women's Ward

"We've been looking for you. You are a silly sausage. It's meds time."

The nurse took her to a line of people. She hoped they would give her Librium; it should have a soporific effect. She'd had it before. It should stop the DT's. Her hands tremored. It didn't help in R's case: her craving for a cigarette was greater. She found her way to the smokers' room because a girl had explained how to get there.

There were boxes she needed to climb over but as she stepped on them, they turned to tiny filaments of colours she had never seen before. She tried to play with them, catch the newness. If she concentrated she could move them and enjoy their unfamiliar tint. She still wanted to see her boxes but thought she might be being observed. She hid her thoughts in her pocket and leant on the wall for some kind of stability.

The next morning she ate her Weetabix, remembered not to tell about her shapes or talk to her cereal.

Half an hour later her Librium thoughts returned to near rationality. She placed her nonconformity and the boxes under the bed where they belonged. Order was important.

She thought she might have been to an interview, there were people in a room, a metal trolley swung sideways and there were people sitting behind large oak desks. Maybe they might have explained why she was there. She wasn't sure.

Someone took out what seemed to be notes from a manila envelope and talked at her.

"Do you understand?"

"Yes," she didn't know what else to say.

"You're free to go then."

R followed a linoleum corridor and saw women sitting in a room, it seemed quiet.

"Can I come in?"

"Yes you daft bat, course you can. Draw up a chair and have a fag, have a Silk Cut, but you'll have to be quick, its meds soon."

"What's that?"

"When you get your tablets."

"Don't have any so far."

"You will have when you're here."

"But I'm not ill, least don't think so."

"Well someone has said you are or you wouldn't be in a mental hospital."

"Is that where I am?"

"Well where do you think you are, the Ritz?"

"Don't really know."

"Right we'd better get there, come on stub it out. You'd better be first in line because you're new."

"Can't any of you get here on time, come on. Move!" the nurse instructed.

The nurse gave R pills in a plastic cup. She swallowed them on the way for a cigarette. She sat down and lit up a JPS. An assistant rushed into the room.

"You know medication has to be supervised."

8

The Women's Ward

"No, I've only just arrived."

"Well that doesn't matter, you should have watched what the other patients did, now give me that tissue paper in your hand!

"I'd rather not, I've got a cold and it's got phlegm on it."

"Don't you try to get clever with me. Now open your mouth so I can look where you've hidden them. Tongue up."

"You have to do as you are told when you are sectioned," a fellow patient interjected. "What do you mean "sectioned"? I'm on detox. Librium four times a day." replied R. "It's the drink that did it."

"Just do as you're asked and take the tablets."

"No, but what do they mean sectioned?"

"Just do as you are told."

R looked across the room and saw a woman who appeared to be smiling in her direction. She had fat blonde hair but fiddled with the tendrils of her hair until they seemed to have changed to a darker shade.

"Come on, I heard what the nurse said, look I'll explain it to you, don't expect you'll like it, but here it goes. They can make you take medication but you can go for a day's leave if you behave yourself and, if you pass your assessment week, they will decide whether you are allowed in the canteen or that kind of thing," explained the woman.

"Sounds awful but they can't keep me here. I've done nothing wrong, just taken a few pills too many. It's really frightening here."

"Well it's not a bundle of laughs. Denise hasn't been outside for a year. I know she's a bitch but you don't wonder she tries to escape. When she succeeds in her flight, her home leave is cancelled and she has to stay in the ward, even for her meals because she's sectioned."

"No one used the word section so I expect I'm not" R responded.

"Lucky you."

R queued watching the wall behind her because she didn't know what else to do. Posters were Blu-tacked in a haphazard way. *We are here to help you. PALS.* A lady smiled benignly from the pamphlet, her hair neatly coiffured.

The poster was couched in short sentences and simple language. R was transfixed by the amount of information.

"Oh, for God's sake, what the hell do you think those pamphlets do for any of us? We're all mad, that's why we're here."

R was fascinated by the myriad cures on the pamphlets, some of which were curled up at the edges and obscured by more recent additions. On the bulletin board one caught her attention. It was written in red on a yellow background and seemed to answer all possible dysfunctions.

Domestic violence, loneliness, gay and lesbian support, sexual abuse, depression, anorexia, bulimia, self-harming and drug-dependency.

The Women's Ward

She chose domestic violence and lesbianism because up until this time she had known nothing about them.

A nurse brought her back from her thoughts.

"We can't wait for ever while you daydream. Come and take your medication or you know what the only other option will be!"

She didn't because she had only been there for a day. The hatch of the dispensary was still open, but the staff were nearing the end of their shift and were becoming short-tempered.

No-one had explained the routines.

She took the paper cup to the smokers' room, swallowed the tablets and was just about to light her first cigarette of the day when an assistant rushed in.

"Right, well let's look at the tissue in your hand. Open your mouth so I can see what's under your tongue. Clever are we? Now, you silly girl, I need to look in your bag because I have reason to believe you have concealed something. Do I have your permission to search you?"

"No."

The assistant ignored R's response, throwing the contents of her bag onto the coffee table and searched the contents for possible hidden pills.

"Right, so you think you're *so* clever, you've managed it this time but don't expect to get away with hiding your pills again. We'll be watching you.

"But I..."

The conversation was closed as the assistant turned her back and walked briskly out of the room.

Most of the other women seemed to be oblivious to the search but a young girl with bright blonde hair and immaculate make-up waved to her.

"Come on, sit here with us."

R was grateful for any kind of invitation and joined the group.

"You're obviously new, you look like a frightened rabbit. I'm Kit by the way, welcome to the nearly normal club. Have a cig."

R wasn't sure how near normality she was but noticed a friendly smile, slightly obscured by long hair which drifted forward over her face.

"Come on we can sort you out, we'll get there or at least somewhere. For the first week, whether voluntary or not, patients have to be assessed on the ward, even what they ate is recorded, attitude to staff noted and social skills monitored to see if they have any." Kit told her the procedures. "Some of the patients," she explained, "have been incarcerated for months and don't breathe fresh air, even though there is a garden totally enclosed by an eight-foot wall. Sorry to sound depressing but that's how it is. Never mind, we have a good laugh sometimes."

The next morning R stumbled through the corridor and noticed sepia pictures, one of which was titled "A Victorian Asylum". Maybe someone

The Women's Ward

had a sense of humour, or perhaps it was an oversight or perhaps it was just an ordinary hospital?

R was afraid she had not wanted to be there in the first place, she had only wanted to die at one moment, die for not being a good enough mother, teacher, wife or person.

The patients were too loud, one was screaming, the others arguing, the staff shouting above the noise. This time she chose the bathroom. It had a lock on the door.

"They can't find me here."

Later the door was unlocked.

"Oh there you are you stupid girl, you know we check where you all are every fifteen minutes. Now you've wasted my time. I have things to do."

"But I didn't know."

"Well you should do. Now get up and come with me."

R only knew that she was afraid but guessed she needed to follow orders. She was led back to her ward.

Later she found her way back to the smokers' room. She stood in the doorway unsure where to sit.

"Come here next to me," Mel suggested.

The ash trays filled up quickly so Kit emptied one for R, rescuing the thin tinfoil receptacle from a chair arm.

"Oh for God's sake you fucking muppet stop crying or they'll section you for sure, think you're suicidal, a danger to yourself" added a large woman.

"But I want to go."

"Don't we all? Just stop that noise: if you sort that out they might let you walk. Listen to Kit, and for God's sake light that fag."

Kath put her arm round R.

"It's nicotine therapy, better than manicure Monday, the only therapy we get."

R didn't understand but accepted the cigarette.

On the next day Kath explained it was review day, that it always happened each Tuesday.

"They decide how ill we are and if we can have home leave. Don't worry about it because the most you can hope for in your first week is to go to the canteen. They even write down what you eat on the ward."

"Will they give me an appointment?"

""No but we all have to go whenever we are called."

"But I don't feel well."

"Don't tell them that for Christ's sake." Kit added.

"So what do I say?"

"Try to act normal."

"How do I do that?"

"If I knew that I'd have been out of here six months ago."

"What time do I go in?"

"You fucking mad or what? You just wait!" Nicky instructed.

"Yes but the staff will give me a time."

"Between twelve and five."

"Is that because I'm new?"

14

The Women's Ward

"No you muppet, that's just how it is. Stop crying for fuck's sake or they'll keep you in, decide you're suicidal, and there's no fucking way out then" Nicky added.

R was called at three. The door to the room had a small embroidered picture, she imagined created by a previous patient, to prove the hospital's success.

A nurse guided her in. R recognised the psychiatrist because she had seen him before but the other five people were unknown to her. Two had A4 folders so she assumed they were students, the others had nothing to distinguish them.

"And how are we today?"

"Not bad."

"So we're not feeling too well?"

She knew she had got it wrong; being obtuse was not a good idea.

There was a silence.

She was surprised to see an exercise bike clothed in bubble-wrap in one corner and a metal trolley rusting beside it; she forgot the advice she had been given and tried to take in her surroundings and the function of the others surrounding her.

"Are you all assessing me?"

"What do you mean by that?"

"Well, it's, nothing, I only thought!"

"Good, so you are beginning to question and move forward."

"No."

"Shall we start again? Can you tell me what date it is?"

"The tenth of the first, two thousand and six."

"Good, well done!"

"I'm not an imbecile?"

"No one is suggesting you are, you are just ill and we are trying to help you."

"Well don't bother!"

She noticed people were taking notes.

"Write this down then, I'm not an exhibit, I'm a person."

She left the room without permission.

The duty nurse caught up with her and R was warned that her behaviour was unacceptable and could result in consequences.

Chapter 2

On the next day Kit explained it was review day, that it always happened each Tuesday,

"They decide how ill we are and if we can have home leave. Don't worry about it because the most you can hope for in your first week is to go to the canteen. They even write down what you eat on the ward."

"Will they give me an appointment?"

""No but we all have to go when they are ready."

"But I don't feel well."

"Don't tell them that for Christ's sake."

"So what do I say?"

"Try to act normal."

"How do I do that?"

"If I knew that I'd have been out of here six months ago."

"What time do I go in?"

"You fucking mad or what, you just wait?" Nicky asked not expecting an answer.

"Yes but the staff will give me a time."

"Between twelve and five."

"Is that because I'm new?"

"No you muppet, that's just how it is. Stop crying for fuck's sake or they'll keep you in; decide you're suicidal and there's no fucking way out then."

The reviews started at twelve. By six o'clock R's anxiety increased and she forgot the advice she had been given.

She had just finished her soup when a nurse called her for the meeting.

The door to the room had a small embroidered picture, she imagined created by a previous patient to prove the hospital's success.

The nurse guided her in.

R recognised the psychiatrist because she had seen him before but the other five people were unknown to her. Two had A4 folders so she assumed they were students, the others had nothing to distinguish them.

"And how are we today?"

"Not bad."

"So we're not feeling too well?"

She knew she had got it wrong. She tried to remember what to say. There was a silence. R glanced around the room again. She was surprised to see an exercise bike clothed in bubble-wrap in one corner and a metal trolley rusting beside it; she forgot the advice she had been given by the others.

"Are you all assessing me?"

"What do you mean by that?"

"Well, it's, nothing, I only thought!"

"Good, so you are beginning to question and move forward."

"No."

"Shall we start again? Can you tell me what date it is?"

"The tenth of the first, two thousand and six."

"Good, well done!"

"I'm not an imbecile?"

18

The Women's Ward

"No one is suggesting you are, you are just ill and we are trying to help you."

"Well don't bother!"

She noticed people were still taking notes.

"Write this down then, I'm not an exhibit, I'm a person."

She left. Maybe she should have listened about how to pretend to be normal.

R felt the need to speak to her husband. Maybe he could sort this mess out.

She went back to her ward and looked in her purse. She found forty pence so located the pay phone. She had now remembered her home telephone number.

It was in a thin grey box; someone had scratched their name on the formica walls and added a date.

She rang but there was no reply so she left a message.

"Hi Dave, the visiting times are 7.30 until 9 o'clock. Can you bring money, cigs and my slippers? Love R."

The money ran out.

She wandered back to the smokers' room and noticed a full packet of cigarettes near to Mel.

"Sorry but will you just lend me a few fags? I'll give them back when my husband visits tonight."

"I suppose so but don't you let me go short."

"No, promise, I've rung him today, so I'm sure he won't forget ciggies."

Mel gave her five, which R tucked into her empty packet.

"Right, thanks, you're a star," R added, "Better go and have a shower and get ready for tonight. Can't wait to see him."

She carefully applied her make-up and changed into a long dress. Dave had told her that her legs were too thin and she was too old to be exposed. He didn't like her to look plain.

She arrived in the lounge at seven in order that she wouldn't miss a second of his time. R picked at the corded edges of the Dralon chair. Waiting.

At seven thirty the visitors arrived but Dave was not among them.

Maybe he was just late; he was never known for his punctuality.

By eight she worried, had he had an accident?

She flicked through a magazine; half looked at the television and for a while watched the others in the room. One had a large bouquet of flowers. Another seemed inundated with chocolate. R seemed to be the only one without a visitor.

R stared at the wall, there was a clock. She became absorbed in its movement. The thick black hands jerked at each minute. The dial was slightly yellowed, there was a scratch, and the enamel had peeled back at nine o'clock. She realised he wasn't coming.

"I expect he's busy what with working full time, housework and cooking. I shouldn't have left him with all that work. If he takes me home everything will be alright."

She delved into what she remembered from her past or what she hoped had been her past.

He would come tomorrow. She would ring her next door neighbour to make sure the message had got through. She had to ask for money and Nicky gave her fifty pence.

"Tell him the phone seems to be out of order but visiting times are from seven until nine. Thanks a lot. See you soon."

The next night R went for a shower to freshen up in preparation for his visit but he didn't arrive.

She was aware that he no longer loved her, if he ever had, but she had had hoped there was a semblance of friendship, if only because of the children, but her faint optimism untangled by nine o'clock. Not even a telephone call. She went back to her ward, hugged her knees to her chest and began to cry. The saltiness covered her cheeks and ran down through her nostrils, meeting with the drops of saliva, which squeezed through the sides of her mouth, in an effort to try not to believe what she knew to be true.

"Right, don't let them see you like this" Nicky admonished.

R left for a moment. She pulled her suitcase from under the bed. It seemed that she would be staying there forever.

Ruth Carter

The clothes were creased but she no longer cared; he had not come to rescue her or even to ask how she was.

R started to reassemble her past. The diary was squashed in the bottom of the clothes. She had hidden it from her husband who discouraged her writing because of, as he explained, the paucity of her intellect. He wasn't there. She was free to write her thoughts. She picked at the curled plastic of the cover but began to write with a blunt pencil.

"Workers
 Drone
Their needs
Pollen driven
Drudgery
We fly
Carrying
A load
Bigger than
Us.
But
I will
Continue
The flight for
Salvation.

The pollen
Is too heavy
I can only
Speak to the summer
And ask for

The Women's Ward

Her help."

Her husband had laughed at her attempts, had encouraged her to be more practical, to hoover, cook and generally to be a wife but she still missed the possibility of some kind of connection.

She lay back in her bed and covered her face in the duvet.

Chapter 3

Thelma stood between the television and the care assistants' afternoon soaps.

She was in the middle of the room, her elasticised floral skirt hitched into her knickers; the jumper had yesterday's breakfast sketched on it.

"Uncomfortable."

She rubbed her crotch, breasts and armpits.

"Uncomfortable."

Even so, staff patted her as they went past, even though she interrupted their television soaps.

They knew her and her need for ECT every three months.

Thelma later she said she had looked forward to it. She would have her words back. Before ECT she only had one word but the staff explained to the others that she would return to near normality as she had the previous times. They were not sure if she understood when they explained she needed to sign a form. It didn't seem to matter in her case. She was deemed incapable of informed consent.

Kit, on the other hand, was apprehensive but she had been told that ECT was the only way to have her children returned. She worried that it wouldn't work, but would have done or have gone through anything to keep her girls, anything to shorten their separation.

Monday morning and they were both tagged "Nil by mouth."

The Women's Ward

There had been an emergency so they waited, dry-mouthed, for three hours.

"How much longer do I have to wait for the electricity? I was scared enough before but I need my family back."

R, the voluntary, offered a coffee, forgetting that Kit couldn't drink.

"I'm not going, I can't stand the waiting. I never wanted it in the first place" Kit complained.

Several patients offered Kit a smoke. Cigarettes at least temporarily calmed her down.

"Nil by mouth," they assumed, didn't include nicotine.

"This waiting around, I was scared enough before, I never wanted this in the first place but they gave me little option, they said it was in my best interest and I suppose they're the experts."

R began to try to orientate herself to the new surroundings and ignore Kit's distress. The walls in the smokers' room had been redecorated because a previous client, she had been told, had set fire to it. The paper was damp through condensation, the windows only opened by about four centimetres (for safety's sake).

Kit was becoming agitated and peeled off a strip of the flowered wallpaper which an ex-client had begun; the other smokers looked at each other.

"The morning cigarette doesn't taste the same without a coffee" Kit complained.

R tried to ignore the yellow tinged walls, especially as she knew she contributed to them, but the butter ochre distracted her from Kit's distress.

"Shit, why did I agree to this? Believe it only works for some; what am I doing? I really don't want to do it. Maybe the treatment is a punishment for all I have done wrong in the past."

R was embarrassed, so turned her attention back to the room. She wondered if the institution would run to replacing the carpet, pebble-dashed with chewing gum, or was it part of their rehabilitation to clean up after themselves? The ingrained ash, which the morning hoover never quite obliterated, remained.

Kit had explained that they were supposed to go at nine o'clock but both waited dry mouthed until nearly twelve.

"Sorry it's a bit late ladies but you know how things go."

Neither of the patients spoke but followed the man down the thin corridor.

Thelma was still "uncomfortable" and Kit in tears brought on by the unknown and the long wait. Kit, being sectioned, was not considered well enough to make "an informed choice."

All she knew was that they could withhold her children if she didn't comply; she was well enough to understand that her sectioning would go up an octave if she refused recommended treatment.

She had smoked about twenty cigarettes between six and twelve.

The Women's Ward

"You will be fine; I've had it twice, it doesn't hurt" Mel tried to reassure Kit. "It didn't work for me but you never know."

At twelve Big John arrived. He was the assistant who was to accompany them to the main hospital for their treatment.

Two hours later they returned. Thelma joined the rest of them in the smokers' room.

"Anyone got a smoke?" she asked. It was the first complete sentence she had uttered.

Kit had gone to her room. R went to visit her but found her comatose and snoring. The duty doctor was called at two o'clock; one of the women overheard the conversation when he was summoned.

"Just a bad reaction to the anaesthetic, she needs to sleep it off. I'll give her something."

The doctor injected her and left.

The next day Kit seemed dazed.

"What happened? Why am I sitting in here? Do I smoke?"

"Yes. Silk Cut, but you can have one of mine" Mel responded.

"Do I have children?"

"Yes, two girls."

"Shit, what are their names?"

"One's called Eve and I think the other one is Helen."

"Well that's a start I suppose."

The following morning they worried about Kit because she didn't appear until after breakfast.

"Where is she, has anybody seen her?"

"No but I expect it was what they gave her last night."

Kit appeared at about ten o'clock.

"I think I'm called Kit; is that right?"

"Yes bloody muppet."

Kit didn't reply, just looked confused.

"Go on then, just have a fag," Nicky suggested.

R, being a voluntary patient, was allowed out after her breakfast and she bought the cigarettes: Super Kings, Richmonds and JPS. She wrote a list and distributed them.

Kit seemed more comfortable later, in the smokers' room, than previously. She didn't have to prove her sanity or disclose where her stash of pills was, she had a scant memory. Really she didn't recall where she had left them. The other women shared her apprehension.

"What happened? Why am I sitting in here? Do I smoke?"

"You usually smoke Silk Cut but you smoked them all yesterday."

"Is it somebody's birthday soon?"

"Yes, your daughter's, on Tuesday."

"Why can't I remember?"

"You ordered her a cake I think" R said.

"Where are they? Should I have done something? Where are they?"

The Women's Ward

"Helen is with your step-dad and Eve with your first husband."

"Did I have two of them, husbands, I mean?"

"Well, so you said, and you've left the second one."

"Do you know why? Because I think he was good at sex. Maybe I have got them muddled."

Thelma spoke; her one previous word had been replaced by a sentence.

"Have you heard about the man who had his legs taken off? He was defeated."

The others laughed in sympathy because of her recovery.

Denise had her music on full blast and tapped her feet frantically, the leather soles slipping on the dais, then whirled into the centre of the room knocking ash trays and coffee mugs onto the floor. Thelma hitched up her skirt and joined in the dancing.

But Kit seemed even more removed.

"Do I smoke? Maybe a cigarette will help."

"Am I really called Kit?"

"Yes you bloody muppet, or we could call you something else, who the fuck do you want to be?"

"I would just like a present or a past."

"Christmas was two weeks ago and at least be fucking glad you can't remember the bad bits. You could always make up a great past. I'd like to forget some of mine"

"Okay, so where am I? Someone explain."

"Have I got a name? Am I real?"

She cried for her lack of being.

R went to get a drink for Kit because she didn't know what else to do. She poured herself a coffee and one for Kit with two sugars.

"Who is the second one for?" asked the assistant.

"For Kit."

"How many times do I have to tell you? Patients get their own drinks, it's part of their recovery process, they need to learn to be self-reliant, fend for themselves."

R tried to remonstrate.

"Well she's ill since her ECT. She's confused."

"That's only temporary, doing little tasks like getting herself a coffee, all those little things are important; as usual you think you know best."

"It's only a coffee, is that detrimental to patients' health?" R retorted.

"Here you go again, always arguing. Her memory loss is only likely to last a few hours and small tasks will help her recovery."

"Fuck you, you have only learned it from text books, you don't live it. We do, we don't do eight hour shifts and go back to our own reality, we have our own which you can't enter even if you wanted to, which I doubt."

R saw the nurse write down something; she thought it might be about her but was too frightened to ask.

"Tell me who I have become or am I just a what?" Kit cried. "Just let me out of here. Just let me out. I promise I will behave. The tablets I keep at home, I promise to tell my husband where my pills are, when I remember. He can bring them in so they know I'm rid of them."

"Oh for God's sake just tell them. Get it over with. They might let you out this side of the century."

Someone else gave Kit another cigarette.

"But really I've forgotten. Do you think we make ourselves sick by the bad things we do or is it just how we are made?

"Don't talk fucking shit" Nicky responded.

R looked on but held Kit's hand, stroked her and tried to stop her picking the hairs off her legs.

Kit, R knew, was sectioned, so had no power to refuse any treatment offered. She was considered too ill to make an informed decision, although the psychiatrist had once tried to explain how the treatment might work, how she might go home earlier. She scribbled her name at the bottom of the page. The doctor had explained that refusal of recommended treatment would up her "Section".

"Hope Kit will be alright, hope it works for her. Had two lots myself and it made me feel worse" Mel remarked, tugging a lock of hair at the side of her face.

"Silly fucking bitch, you could have told her before she went down" Nicky interrupted.

"Why didn't you warn her Mel? It didn't work for you and you've had ECT twice: you should have warned her" added R.

"But she has no choice if she's sectioned."

"Yes she did, you have to sign a form" added Nicky.

"Tell me again, tell me my name."

Kit's head rested on the side of the chair. She dribbled a little as she slumped down, her eyes were squeezed shut in an attempt to keep the tears at bay. "Am I?"

"Yes honestly."

"Really?"

Mel fiddled with her hair again, twisting it round her index finger in a regular rhythm. Denise tried to join in the conversation, picking up the dog-ends to roll up a new cigarette.

"She was a slapper, anyone's. I know her sort." Denise muttered.

She made her own type of cigarette; she knew the nurses wouldn't intervene because she was calmer afterwards. It was simpler to ignore her lack of regulation.

She was considered too ill to go to the café or walk in the gardens. She needed to be constrained but her spliffs were tolerated. She was a danger. It was not clear to whom, maybe to society in general or to herself, but she had been denied fresh air for the length of her internment. When her boyfriend arrived, they sat with legs akimbo, she leant into his crotch and began licking his trousers to his obvious enjoyment. The other women turned their chairs around in a circle so as not to watch the spectacle; it was not an act they felt should be public, and they had been denied normal contact since their incarceration.

The Women's Ward

After he left, she rolled her spliffs, eight in all. The smokers' room became more fume-ridden than usual. One of the group complained to the office because she had become befuddled with the smoke. No-one listened. Vodka and dope calmed her and she was not such a problem as usual.

There was an official complaint from the body of the women; they were denied sex themselves and saw no reason why she should be an exception. That resulted in the boyfriend being instructed not to enter the smokers' room; the couple resorted to the room designated as a gym, although it only had three plastic covered mats on the floor, but it was at least private, the cameras had not yet been installed.

Nicky sat back down and lit up, regaining her composure. She looked at R's feet.

"Right your shoes look as big as mine; can I borrow your shoes for tomorrow?"

Nicky was persuasive.

"Go on then, but you will need to de-smell them because I've got athletes foot."

"Sod that, if you've got fucking hepatitis, I still need them."

"Okay you silly bitch have them."

The afternoon had been difficult; R tried to explain herself so she might exist.

She had ideas above her station; her husband always reminded her of that. She had once tried to write, like Sylvia Plath, but could only think of the intricacies of flies' eyes. It would hardly be a popular subject because they have dirty feet and contaminate food. Only the nurses were allowed sprays; they used them to eliminate any contamination on the wards.

Her psychiatrist had tried his best to order her; saw her as a hawk moth rather than the butterfly she hoped to be.

"Don't logic me, I am an enigma" she tried to explain but nobody listened.

"I would rather be a mayfly, just a few hours of life and disappear, just one day, it would be enough. Ordinary people don't understand they are removed from my kind of unreality. Yes, I realised, I played a game, nearly knew how to escape. It was "The Glass Bead Game" but I never got past the introduction."

She tried to explain herself. R would have liked to explain the Chicken Lickiness of her state of not being but knew that to mention it to staff would only extend her stay. She tried to explain it to the women.

"Shut up, you are getting to my tits. Just because you are the odd one doesn't give you the right to talk shit."

In the morning they looked at the board to see which staff were on. Apart from the dark haired one who did "Manicure Mondays," the rest were wonderful, but some of the night nurses were feared, with the exception of Gwen who loved even the most disturbed, who held them through their insanity.

The Women's Ward

"Come on, you will get there, even though you are unsure at the moment. Just believe me." They loved Gwen, but the others were sadistic, Mel explained.

The staffing board explained how the night would be.

Chapter 4

She found her diary; several pages were as blank as she was. She had hidden it deep in the case. Her husband discouraged her writing, explaining that due to her lack of intellect, writing poetry was an anathema; for the first time she ignored him, escaping into her own unreality.

It was a bland day, she watched the fog hug the ground, birds seemed to have forgotten their morning, stars were obscured, no-one, nothing, seemed to be near.

She fingered the dented plastic of her file, ripping the edge away to reveal the cardboard. She opened the first page,

The Happy Reaper.

Please do
Not come to me
When I am asleep.
I would like to have
A conversation with
You, however short.

Do you have job satisfaction?
What is it like to be immortal?
Why do you carry a scythe?
It seems an unnecessary indulgence.
The cloak
Too obviously Gothic.

If I keep awake

The Women's Ward

Maybe we could
Have a conversation.

Do you enjoy your work?
Get job satisfaction?
Was this
Your chosen career?
Wouldn't you have preferred
To be a priest
Or politician?
Impress with your rhetoric?

I could make you a cup of tea.
Do you want sugar?

You don't answer. You will come
With no explanation.

She was glad he hadn't read it; he would only have laughed at her paucity of intellectual capacity. R was imprisoned but free. She wandered to the smokers' room in the hope of some company. She brought her book with her in an attempt to hold her thoughts together. She sat in the only free chair; it was in the corner which pleased her because she could hide herself. She began to write again for comfort and the hope that she could begin to understand.

Silence
Holds
My mortality

Ruth Carter

Crows
Caw my
Death
They feather
Me with their darkness.
But the iridescence
Is
My nearest
Rainbow.

A woman interrupted her writing.

"Why the fuck do you keep scribbling? Aren't we good enough to talk to?"

"Sorry, just trying to sort my head out."

"Well for God's sake don't let the staff see it unless it's positive. They go through your stuff to look at your mood, they'll keep you in for sure if you sound depressive."

"But they wouldn't go through my diary!"

"In your dreams; everything is searched. Can tell you're new."

R put down her book.

"But that would be a breach of civil liberties."

"We don't have any of those in here. Not even allowed out for exercise unless you are thought emotionally fit to breathe fresh air. Break one rule, however small, and you are kept on ward arrest."

"But it's a hospital not a prison."

"So you think," the woman added. "Look, just do as you're told, keep looking happy. We're monitored by CCTV, they write down everything we do."

"They sound like the thought police; it can't be true."

"Believe me it is. At least you seem to be getting the picture. Just put that bloody book down. I'll grab you a coffee and put some music on. I'm June by the way."

"I'm R."

"That's not a name, it's an initial. No wonder they keep you in here, you're just a nutter."

June strode over to the CD player and put on a sixties soul band.

"Back in a minute and do cheer up."

She arrived back two minutes later with a plate of toast and two cups of coffee but she tripped on the curled carpet and spilled one of the drinks down her white skirt. The hot liquid screamed down to her left foot.

"Oh sod it."

She pulled up her skirt and removed her tights to review the damage. There were circles of redness, she kicked off her left shoe to empty out the residue.

"So sorry, sorry. Can I get a nurse to put ointment on it?"

"Don't be; if I tell them they will only think I've self-harmed and keep me in for longer."

"No, they have a duty of care."

June ran her finger nails along the aluminium frame of the window, it screeched her frustration.

"Sorry, have I made you cross?" asked R.

"And you can stop bloody apologising. It was just an accident. You couldn't help ruining my best skirt. The top's buggered as well. Seems to me every time I try to do a favour, I bollocks up."

R noticed the stains had begun to solidify. June plonked the remaining half cup of coffee on the rough surface of the small Formica table top.

"No you have it, really. I'm not thirsty."

"Just drink it and shut up. I'll have to go and clean my clothes. I just hope it dries by tomorrow, it's my interview, my only chance of escaping. Just have your fucking coffee."

"No really, you have it."

"You fucking drink it."

Both women sat in their separate silences after the exchange. The other women continued their conversations.

"Come on girls, it's tea time, let's get a move on, you don't want it to get cold," Shaun told them.

"But I'm not hungry," R replied to the nurse.

"It's part of your therapy."

"Oh so I have to get fat to be happy?"

"Come on, the food's good. Just try it."

"Don't know I have a choice. Have to do as I'm told. I've learned that much."

She joined the queue waiting for the door to be unlocked so that they could go to the cafeteria.

The Women's Ward

"Okay," John explained, "It's your first day at the café so I'll take you down. I can make sure you're safe."

"So what do you think I'd do, throw myself down the stairs or something, or start to bite people?"

"It's been known."

He held her arm as they descended the stairs. There were men seated at tables, she had not interacted with such creatures for some time. Dave still didn't visit and there were normally only men there who were paid to administer palliative care.

Alan was one of those assistants who R thought she related to. He talked to her about his family, his training and aspirations; he seemed to seek her out to share his philosophies and their mutual beliefs.

As a voluntary patient R was allowed out for six hours a day provided she returned for meals. That day she had been asked by Kit to buy some new clothes for her. She had put on a stone in two weeks, Olanzapine made her constantly hungry.

"Get me ten Mars bars and a few Snickers bars."

"No chance, I'll get you clothes that will fit you. Don't worry about the money, you can pay me when you get your benefits."

"Come on. Do me a favour, I've no money left. Can't even buy cigs or a chocolate bar."

"Clothes first, cigs second and one chocolate bar."

R spent her outside time in charity shops and came back laden with shopping for those who were not allowed out.

She was let in.

"Good shop then?" Alan asked.

"Yes, think I've got everything."

"Let's see what you've bought then."

"No you wouldn't want to know. It's only second hand clothes and a Mars Bar for Kath."

Alan followed her into her ward.

"Sorry about this but I need to look through your shopping."

"Why? Don't you trust me?"

"It's not like that, just in case you've brought something in by accident which could cause you or the other patients harm."

"I've read the list of what's allowed or not. Do you think I'm stupid or what? Oh sorry that goes without saying in this place. Sorry, I thought you were kind of a friend. Shouldn't get ideas above my station, after all I'm just a mad person."

"No it's just that I'm on SAS duty."

"Suddenly joined the army then?"

"No, it's Safety and Security." Alan replied as he tipped the contents of her carrier bags onto the bed.

The Women's Ward

"Better look through my handbag and pockets. Could be anything there, vodka, needles, pins, biros or the odd spliff. Just anything."

"Come on, we don't need to go that far," he said trying to calm her or so he hoped.

R tipped the contents of her handbag onto the bedside table. Old sweets and a moisturiser rolled onto the floor.

"When you've finished at least fold them up. Go on keep looking. You won't find anything."

"Didn't think I would."

"So what's with the search? Just rip apart what I stupidly thought was some kind of rapport. Must have been a real idiot to think you actually respected me."

"Don't get upset."

"Right, get a female member of staff to strip search me! Might as well go for it, let's stick to the rules."

"Come on, you know are things are."

"Yes, too bloody well. How come no-one searches Denise's boyfriend when we know he brings in vodka and spliffs? That's it!" she said, throwing her jacket on the floor. "Don't worry, my trousers don't have pockets, catch up with me later if you want to check."

Kit came over and put her arm on R's shoulder.

"Believe me, you just have to ride with it."

R left her ward and fled to the smokers' room.

Ann was standing in the centre.

43

"Hi R, just a question for you. Have you ever thought about the difference between men and women?"

"No not really," R said wiping her nose with her sleeve. "Don't give a shit. They're all bastards."

"No, listen. Why do men have to stand up to have a piss, then shake it so it dribbles on the carpet? Why don't they sit down and use toilet roll like we do?" Ann asked.

R began to giggle. She hadn't thought of that before, men were an anathema, especially her husband.

Chapter 5

It was just before breakfast when Wiggy arrived in the room.

"Anyone lend me a fag?" she asked.

R gave her a JPS.

"Sorry but Pete didn't arrive yesterday."

"Who's he then?" R asked.

"He looks after my benefit book so it doesn't get stolen. He does it for lots of us. He's dead kind that way."

"Go on, you plonker, don't expect he does it for love. What's in it for him?" Nicky asked.

"Well he does take a bit for his troubles."

"Go on then, how much?" Nicky enquired, straightening her dressing gown.

"Go on Wiggy, spit it out."

Nicky pretended to yawn and looked up to the ceiling.

"Come on, give."

"Well, fifteen pounds."

"What? A week?"

"Well yes, but he looks after me."

"He's a loan shark," R remarked.

"What's one of those then?" Wiggy asked.

"It's someone who rips people off, steals their money. I hate men like that. They're just greedy bastards. Get rid Wiggy, he's bad news" rasped Nicky. "You're more stupid than I took you for and that's saying something."

Wiggy clasped her hands together and rubbed the cheap ring on her forefinger. She wriggled down in the chair and stared at her feet.

"No, you don't understand, he's a friend, really he is. He helps loads of us. Even has other people to help him. They go to the offices. All you have to do is just sign, dead easy."

"Just get your book sent to the hospital, they'll sort the money out," R said.

"That is if it doesn't get lost in the administration. Everything in this place seems to get lost in red tape." Nicky added.

"Come on don't be such a cynic" R remonstrated.

"You know she's such a silly bitch, she won't listen even in her lucid moments."

Wiggy began to sniff back tears.

Nicky had rolled up her sleeves and began picking at the large scab under her left elbow. The blood streaked down to her hand.

R decided to try and change the subject but was unsure what direction to go in. She was embarrassed by Nicky's obvious distress and it clouded her judgement.

"How did your arms get hurt?"

"The cat scratched them. What do you think? Don't be so fucking nosey!" She responded, trying to pull her sleeves down to disguise the damage.

"No, I thought you might have had an accident, that's all" R added lamely.

The Women's Ward

"You're the fucking accident, motor mouth. No I didn't" she answered, pulling herself and lumbering over to R.

R clutched the frayed covering of her chair, her fingers met with the escaping foam which she hoped might distract her from the probable assault.

"Okay, if you must know, not that it's your bloody business, but I used a scrubbing brush to make sure the caustic soda went into my skin. It turned septic. Satisfied now? Who do you think you are? The Gestapo?"

"Sorry, didn't realise."

"Well think next time."

R offered a cigarette.

"Just sod off."

Nicky pulled up her long velvet skirt and stared at R before leaving the room.

R followed her into the lounge to apologise.

"Sorry I didn't mean to offend."

Nicky pressed the volume control on the television remote and turned her back on R, shoulders hunched.

R retreated, returning to the smokers' room.

Wiggy was sitting on a chair opposite to the door and almost seemed to be smiling.

"Sorry I shout sometimes, but I only do it in my own room, it's not at any of you lot. Just shouting at things in my past. Things I should have said, told the bastard. Kicked me in the stomach, got rid of the kid he didn't want. Keep thinking, what if I had stood up to him? Too late now. That's why I want a baby now."

Nicky returned because she needed another cigarette but she ignored R.

"Think it's a bit late. Going to be the oldest mother in the world?" Nicky replied. "They do it in Tibet, maybe you could get one of those woollen helmet things with sort of strings, could increase your fertility."

"God knows what programme you watched. Believe me it's too late for both of us."

R tried to retrieve her previous conversation with Nicky.

"That's a nice blouse."

"Same one I had on this morning."

"Sorry must not have noticed."

"No, you never do."

They were distracted by Wiggy who opened a carrier bag onto the floor.

"Look what I got today. I was allowed out with a nurse and bought some clothes. I'll go and try them on and show you."

She strode into the room minutes later. She was wearing a long silk skirt with a matching jacket and a wide brimmed hat with a plume of feathers at the front.

"Oh gawd, going to a wedding or something," Nicky remarked.

"No, come on you look stunning. If you just pushed your wig back so it doesn't cover your eyes, you'll look stunning," R countered.

"Yes and I might just put on a bit of lippy to wow them at my review next Tuesday."

The Women's Ward

She strode back to her room which was a single. R had heard that Wiggy was considered to be too disturbed to share. Alan had told her.

"My," R whispered, "she seems like the ticket today."

"You just wait until review day," Nicky said chewing her pencil. "Just you watch her wind up. They usually leave her until last. Don't know why because she's a basket case by six."

"So why don't they put her in first? The staff must have noticed."

"You really don't understand. She's long term. Invisible. That's just how it is and anyway we all have to wait from twelve, maybe as long as until six, so why should she be any different?"

"But surely she's ill; they need to take that into account."

"Look, stop asking stupid questions, we're all supposed to be ill." Nicky added. "You'll get yourself in deep shit if you ask why things happen. Come on, I'll give you some of my chocolate if you just shut up."

R tried to understand the rules but was still confused. The chocolate at least distracted her for the moment. She took the wrapper and placed it in the plastic bin. She noticed there were holes in the side where people had stubbed their cigarettes out but the inside of the receptacle was even worse. The bottom was covered in a green slime with decayed objects immersed in it. There was a fetid smell.

"Oh my God. I thought we had cleaners." R complained.

"Not again you silly bitch. Just get used to things."

R gave in and retreated to her ward, pulled the covers up to her chin and began to doze but was quickly woken by a loud noise.

"Look at you filthy girl, you've still got your clothes on."

"But I only came for a lie down because I was upset."

"You can be upset standing up just as well. Now get out of bed, have a bath and put some new clothes on. Even if you are supposed to be ill you can at least be clean. No excuses now, you have wasted enough of my time. Move it. I've already recorded your behaviour on the chart. I don't expect you will want me to write anymore negative comments. It is review date tomorrow and what we say counts," Sarah the assistant added.

"One, two, three," R responded.

"That's it. Think you're clever. That's your home leave gone for the next week."

"Bitch," R muttered but was heard by Sarah. She smiled. "I knew I'd have you one day. Verbal aggression towards a member of staff. Think your so clever being a teacher and all. I didn't get any exams but look where I am now."

"A damn sight more idiotic and sadistic than the patients. Stupidity isn't an excuse for the way you behave. Some of the kindest pupils I have taught have had academic special needs but really cared, which is more than can be said for you. Wouldn't be surprised if you got this job because they don't ask for qualifications and have to take on any scum they can get," R railed, having totally lost her temper and forgotten Nicky's advice.

There was silence for a few seconds as the women observed each other. A tea trolley rattled past the open door.

"Come on you lot, time for tea and biscuits."

Much to R's surprise Sarah sat on the edge of her thin grey duvet and began to chew her nails, lips quivering.

"You didn't need to be so rude. Okay I know I'm a failure. Mum and Dad always said I'd make nothing of myself and my supervisor says I'm too soft with the patients."

R immediately regretted her outburst.

"Look, I'm sorry. I was just a bit upset and you took the brunt. Don't listen to what other people say. You'll do fine."

R propped herself up on the stained pillowcase. Patients were supposed to change their own beds but there was rarely enough linen to go round. She apologised for the state of her bed linen.

"No at least you're your locker top is tidy," Sarah said, trying to retrieve the situation.

"You really are a good girl," R remarked. "Don't let them put you down."

They hugged in their understanding of their mutual needs but were caught by a passing nurse.

"Physical contact between staff or patients is prohibited for obvious reasons. You, Sarah, will be suspended!"

R wanted to respond but knew it was pointless.

On the following Tuesday Wiggy sat with R for breakfast. She had baked beans on toast but used a spoon to eat.

"What about the toast."

"Well I'll just leave it; don't want to spoil my clothes. If I look smart they might let me out for a day or two.

The day seemed to linger; by five Wiggy had not been called. She sat with the others and began to sing quietly with the sixties DVD.

"They've got to let me out. I'm fine. You lot tell them."

"Some fucking chance they would listen to us nutters," Nicky responded.

"We could try. Wiggy is fine until she winds up but they only see her at her bad times," Nicky added.

Wiggy stubbed out a half-smoked cigarette and returned to her room.

The others could hear her grief. The noise permeated the smokers' room.

"You bastard. You threw me down the stairs, kicked me in the stomach, laughing. Bastard. No more baby. Sod off! You caused it all. Bugger, big bugger." she yelled. "Why did they believe you when you said I just fell? It's because of you I've been sectioned. Sod you."

The women could hear her kicking the door and she began to scream.

"Bloody hell, what's changed?" R asked.

The Women's Ward

"It's always like that on a Tuesday when she has to wait for her review. They always seem to leave her until last."

"Well why don't the staff put her in early if she gets so upset?" R remarked.

"Tell you're new. Look, she's long term, staff don't notice her anymore," Mel concluded.
Mel went to Wiggy's room and managed to calm her.

"Shush, the staff will hear you and take your day leave away. Come on, have a fag, I'll give you one." Wiggy followed Mel into the smokers' room.

"Go on one of you, lend us a few fags. He didn't arrive today."

"So who is he?"

She had told them about her friend Peter who brought her cash on a Wednesday and looked after her money as he did for lots of people. He only took twenty for his outgoings she explained.

Zelda was scrunched up behind a chair and the fan which didn't work, it was her usual spot. She had gained her own space. Her short dark hair was plaited and beaded in an approximation of dreadlocks, her eyes swallowed by thick kohl which was accentuated by a thick pale foundation.

She took three steps forward towards the ward, two to the left and one to the right but managed to avoid the walls as she travelled towards the women's room. She spoke to no-one, unless she needed a cigarette, curled up in her own solitude. Some of the staff tried to entice her to speak by promises of a walk in the garden, joining the others for lunch or the possibility of a few hours leave.

She remained mute.

R guessed the girl to be about seventeen and probably autistic, but she tried to reason that the staff would have recognised the symptoms and put her in palliative care.

Although she had taught autistic pupils, and researched possible ways of remediation and had had some measure of success, she did not dare to express her views in case she was seen as interfering with hospital routine. After all it seemed that she had to remember to be a patient. She had been admonished in the past when she had hugged the Filipino girl who was begging to die.

"So you are at it again, getting too close. Physical contact between patients is not allowed. You never know what it might lead too," the assistant remarked. She wrote something down on her chart.

"Don't worry, I've recorded your behaviour," she continued, "All your actions will be fed back in your review and you know what that means, no weekend leave for you." The woman ticked several boxes and left.

Maybe she could explain to Sean. She could voice her concerns about Zelda's mechanical movements in the corridor, always three steps forward, two to the right, then two to the left. The pattern continued until she reached the room. She never made eye contact but shuffled into the place the other women had cleared for her, all typical behaviour of the autistic pupils R had taught in her previous life, but surely, she reasoned, the staff must have noticed, but maybe the condition did not come under the umbrella of mental health. R decided against mentioning her idea to a member of staff. She was learning to be silent. Instead she took out her last cigarette and gave it to the girl.

R looked out of the window again, waiting for the rain, annoyed that she was too afraid to speak. Any observation would be recorded as interference.

"Come on, you bloody daydreaming again," laughed Nicky.

"Just thinking," R answered.

"Well don't bother. It's not encouraged in here and anyway it will probably give you a headache. Come on, get a grip, it's nearly time for lunch!"

R really didn't feel like eating but was learning about the regime; eating was carefully monitored, consumption recorded and used as a measure of mental health. She could not afford to be written up as depressive.

She queued up with the others and looked at the menu, blue-tacked to the café door.

Roast pork

Roast beef

Vegetable stew

Mel was in front of her in the line. They were both a little late because R waited for her friend who was looking for a stray false nail.

The roast beef was finished but there was a pile of left-over Yorkshire puddings.

"Right you two, get a move on. It's not the Hilton," the young girl admonished.

"Okay, I'll have Yorkshire puddings, pork, green beans and roast potatoes."

"Don't be silly, normal people only eat Yorkshire's with beef,"

"Well that's why I'm in here, not quite the ticket. Now can I have my food?"

"For God's sake be quiet or you will get yourself reported" Mel said.

"She's only a kid," R responded.

"We shut in two minutes, so just get a move on or you'll get nothing."

Mel opted for the vegetable stew although it was a little congealed. R was incensed.

"Two Yorkshires and the left over beef stock."

The girl picked up the gravy and poured it in the slops.

"That's not allowed young lady, have a proper meal."

"Don't you "Young lady" me. I'm old enough to be your grandmother."

"Right I'll report you. What's your name?"

"Rasputin," R replied.

The girl seemed confused so continued her cleaning. R helped herself to a cup of tea and a biscuit.

"Don't give me a load of grief, you're all of eighteen, younger than my son."

The Women's Ward

"Look I've been trained, went to college and everything."

"What, how to make overcooked vegetables and be offensive?"

"No need to be rude."

"Patronising bitch," R muttered losing her temper. The girl pushed down the shutters. An assistant came up.

"If you don't calm down I'll have to write an incident form."

Nicky reappeared, behind R.

"Don't you ever do as you are told? Don't you ever learn? Just conform."

"Bollocks, she's only a kid. I'm not taking that shit from her."

"I know the ropes."

"Go on then, they've kept you in for a year, sounds more like string than a rope. Pretty long learning curve," R snapped.

"Just sit still and calm down!"

Nicky left her chair and wrapped her ample arms around R. She picked up her own tray and deposited it on the trolley before opening the door with a scratched label with "Private" marked in red.

She reappeared with the left-overs of the vegetable stew, grease-ridden and sodden.

"Sorry, best I could do. Come on eat up."

"But they are all mushy, someone has let the vitamins escape," R added.

"Good, at least the canteen hasn't canned your sense of humour."

R pushed the vegetables around her plate but knew she had to be seen to eat something.

They were the last ones eating and John sat with them.

"Not hungry then? Feeling a bit down?"

"No, just understand why you assistants get take-aways."

"Staff are not allowed to eat hospital food."

"That's because it's such crap. Only fit for patients," Nicky interposed.

Trying to defuse the situation John tried to change the subject.

"Come on you two, it's a lovely day. The sun is shining, it's a lovely day."

"Would be nice if you lot ever let me out," retorted Nicky, appearing to try to rub off the faded tattoo on her right arm in anger.

"Don't worry, we will let you out when you are well enough."

"Says who?"

He did not reply.

The assistant had observed the altercation in the café and was trying to put things right, maybe because he was waiting for his own lunch break.

"Look," he said stroking invisible creases in his T-Shirt, "Just calm down, go to your room and I'll bring you a sandwich."

"What, one of the curled-up ones?"

"You have to eat something to improve."

"Who says so? The food police?"

John looked at the clock, twenty past one. The girl in the café collected R's uneaten dinner.

"I'd like a sandwich for my little friend," the assistant asked.

The Women's Ward

"We don't serve food after one."

"Just a sandwich."

"I'm off duty now, so if you wouldn't mind moving."

John touched R's arm.

"Come on you, I'll sneak off to the chippie and buy you something but in return you have to promise not to cry otherwise I won't let you have the ketchup from the kitchen."

R smiled for the first day in weeks.

"Right girls if you're ready, up the apples and pears."

"Patronising git," Nicky remarked in a whisper.

"No, but he often treats me as a person, or at least he used to."

John picked at the side of his moustache and fiddled with the edge of his cuff.

"Come on ladies."

"You still have a lot to learn, we come in as a bad second, being mad" Nicky added.

"But John's okay, he's nice to me."

"Don't be fooled, he's still part of the system."

The girl reappeared with a mop and bucket and cleaned noisily, tutting as she mopped under their feet.

"Come on you lot, just move, I do have a job to do. Just go, or I'll have to report you for not following orders."

"Wait a minute, I'm a member of staff," he said fiddling with his plastic identity card.

"Sorry didn't realise, I thought you were one of them," she spluttered.

The women moved reluctantly. They picked their way through left-over containers and Coke bottles which had been discarded.

Chapter 6

Ann rushed in, pivoting in front of the television.

"Mad as a fish cake or a tin of baked beans, they wouldn't let them out on their own. Maybe that's why I'm still here," she explained.

"You see I know what's what or what I should be, you could paint me. Make me into a saint and put my statue into a church, someone might throw holy water on me or light candles as a beatitude."

R walked slowly towards her and took her by the hand.

"Come on, sit next to me, we can watch the telly.

Ann rested her head on R's shoulder, R stroked her hair and Ann fell asleep. There were no staff available because it was change over time when paper work had to be shared and duplicated. Only an emergency bell could move them.

It was a time for staff not to have to try to interact with patients. Nurses usually had a coffee and cake at this point.

Ten minutes after the meeting finished Alan appeared in the lounge.

"I was looking out the window during our talk. I saw what you did for Ann, you should be a member of staff not a patient."

"Yeah, I could do with just doing an eight hour shift. Hope that was a compliment any how."

"You know we get on well. Why would I be rude to you?"

"You usually are," R laughed.

Ann continued her contribution, rubbing her eyes to disperse the pus in the corners and standing up to address her audience.

She pirouetted; the long skirt slapped her legs as she moved.

"I'm one of the million millipedes, I've just lost a leg, not that you lot would have noticed, but it was number seventy-five and I miss it. You might think I'm silly but I'm as normal as the rest of you. I watch Brookside and Eastenders."

She plonked down in her chair, folded a soggy tissue in her hand and giggled.

"You lot think I'm crackers, but I'm not Jacob's, probably a cheap packet from Morrison's for ten pence. Never was one to spend too much."

R held her hand because she had become shaky. Sarah the assistant walked in briskly.

"You can stop that silliness right now. Go and do something useful for once. Round up the others from the smoker's room, it's the meeting in five minutes."

R did as she was told; she had become used to obeying orders.

They took up their allotted positions in the velour-covered chairs, arranged against the back wall. Unusually the desk was covered in a

The Women's Ward

tablecloth and there was a bottle of Perrier water and a glass.

Sarah reappeared bringing somebody in with her; she was on duty that day. She stood behind the desk and straightened the creases on her top.

"Right ladies, we have a guest speaker today. He's called Darren and he's here to explain what occupational therapy has to offer you."

The man had a scrunch of ginger hair and a hint of a beard. He sat down, coughed a little and glanced at his notes on the clip board and took out a marker pen; arranged the flip chart to give it a clean sheet.

"Hi, some of you won't know me, I'm Darren. In charge of the facility, and it's my job to tell you what we can do for you. Right then, cookery, gymnastics, pottery, gardening, how to use a PC, all the life skills which will help you adjust when you get out. It's not just about enjoying yourselves, we help you change; learn what you need to know about the outside world and that kind of thing."

He crossed his corduroyed trousers and shuffled towards his audience on the edge of his chair.

"Any questions so far?"

"What about child care?" asked Wiggy who was patently beyond an age to bear children.

"Well not at the moment."

"But I'm pregnant, what are you going to do about that?"

"We'll look into it."

"You, you're as stupid as a scone."

Wiggy slumped back in her chair and closed her eyes.

"Next, any other queries?"

"Last time you taught me to make beans on toast, really useful that, I can actually open a can!" Nicky interposed, "Got anything a bit more useful this time?"

"Well we all come in at different levels; we cater for that, set the task according to the patient's needs."

"Quite fancied cordon blue actually."

He raised an eyebrow and smiled vaguely in her direction.

"Just pop your idea on the form I'll give you at the end of the session. Okay?"

"I've been waiting for three months for a course, not a sausage," said Babs.

"Well maybe you weren't well enough; we do take advice from your nurses."

"Oh I see, you have to be well before therapy."

The volume had been turned off but the television still flickered in the corner, some of the women tried to decipher morning television with no sound. Mel shuffled her feet on the worn carpet and stared at the rain splattered window. She noticed that the blinds had not been mended, the one on the right tilted and the others had large grey threads hanging from them.

Darren shifted a little and tugged at a piece of hair which fell over his forehead.

"Back to business. As I was saying, we have lots to offer, all you need to do is fill in these forms."

The Women's Ward

Sarah stood up.

"Right, well thank you for your input, I'm sure we have all learned a lot, haven't we ladies?"

"Bollocks."

"No need to be rude Nicky."

Darren shook hands with a few of the more acquiescent patients then filled in the paper work at the desk.

The other women left but R stayed, now the Librium had worn off she could get her bearings. Was the television bolted down to stop it being stolen or because a patient she had never met might become violent and try to throw it across the room?

There was a large collage, tinselled round the edges, with cotton-woolled Father Christmases, there were remnants of tissue paper and deflated balloons. It was August, or at least she believed it was but in there it still seemed to be winter.

The man walked across to her and placed a hand on her shoulder.

"Still thinking of what course to take then?"

"No not really, just don't know where I am or where the lessons are."

"It's easy, just down the corridor, expect there'll be an escort to show you the way."

"Thanks."

"See you soon then."

He collected his paper work and pressed the buttons at the door for his escape.

R cried for want of being and switched the volume up on the television. She knew how to make beans on toast but she filled in the forms for want of anything better to do. Ann began to cry so R held her, rocking her gently.

"Sod the rules."

It was a rare moment of rebellion.

"At it again? When will you learn to mind your own business? We know what we are doing. We're trained to look after the likes of her. Just remember that you are only a patient not a member of staff. Go away and behave yourself."

R disentangled herself and in a small act of defiance kissed Ann on the cheek before leaving.

She went to the ward but it was lonely. Dave still hadn't called. There was nothing on the answer phone. She decided to take her one cigarette to the room, she would save the second half for later but she decided to take her diary with her to explain to herself what she was thinking.

"What the fuck do you think you are doing?" asked Nicky. "Better go and get rid of that stain on your jumper. They notice that kind of thing. Lack of self-care. You might have been a teacher but for God's sake stop scribbling or they'll keep you in for sure."

Nicky squashed her cigarette on the tinfoil holder but it tipped over leaving the remnants on the chewing-gummed floor. She scrubbed the remains into the carpet but retrieved the stubs and placed them in the bin. She brushed the ash from her velvet skirt.

The Women's Ward

"Bollocks, you made me do that, your writing all the time does my head in. Are you not quite the ticket? Mind you, expect you wouldn't be here if you were the ticket."

She shook her head and lit up another cigarette.

"Bollocks, why should I put up with the likes of you? All books but no conversation. Just fuck off and bury yourself in a book, or in your case maybe it needs to be a library."

"No need to be rude."

"Why not?"

"Well I need to read and write to see who I am."

"I'll tell you, give that arsehole of a husband the boot. I kicked mine out years ago. Best thing I ever did."

R placed her book on the edge of the coffee table and looked across towards Nicky.

"Never really thought about it."

Nicky wiped the spilt butter from her toast into the creases of her skirt and licked up the remainder with her fingers.

"Trouble with you," she said, "You read so much you don't see how life is. Books and writing just scramble your brains."

R said nothing but did not pick up her book again. The tinfoil shallow ashtrays were usually balanced on the thin wooden arms of the chairs, the coffee tables too far away for easy reach so they spilled the ash on the floor.

They had found healing amongst themselves. The hospital therapy only extended to

"Manicure Monday" when the patients could have their nails painted. Most of them stayed in the smoker's room chewing their nails to the quick. R began to cry because she realised she had upset Nicky.

"Come on you fucking muppet, stop crying and have a fag."

"No that's not enough, I need my tablets."

"Bollocks, what you need is a coffee and a real cigarette, not a roll up from the fag ends. Get a grip; don't let them see you like this."

"Like what?"

"Crying, they'll think you're suicidal, a danger to yourself."

"I just miss my children."

"That won't work, you're monitored, and they watch you."

"But I want to go home."

"If you sort yourself out you can walk, just wait until the end of this week of assessment, if you behave you'll be able to go to the canteen. Okay to start with you'll have a minder, but they don't sit with you. Odd that because if you wanted you could hide a knife and sharpen it if you really wanted to. Becky did it, used the metal end of her bed to hone it and slit her wrists. I suppose if you really want to do it nobody can stop you..."

"Give me a cig, I'll pay you back," Becky asked.

"What like the last three times?"

"Well my giro was late."

The Women's Ward

"What for three weeks running? I'd speak to your social worker about that but the answer is still no."

"What about the Rizla's you stole off Emily last night? You could use the butt ends," added Mel. "I'm not subbing you again."

"She's just a low-life, don't give her anything! She's a taker" said Denise.

Nicky used a tissue to dab off the ash on the arm of her chair.

"Some people are filthy bitches."

She rolled up the thin fabric of her blouse revealing the full glory of her tattooed arms. The word Sarah seemed to have a space of its own, just on the top of her shoulder.

"Who's Sarah?" R asked.

"My daughter, she died in a hit and run accident."

"Sorry, didn't mean to intrude."

Denise stopped her foot tapping and leapt to her feet, she kissed the "Sarah".

"Die you bitch," she screamed as she kissed the name on Nicky' shoulder.

There was a silence.

Nicky gripped the arms of her chair and stood up.

"Right you cow I'll have you for that"

She lumbered over to Denise.

"I'll give you a good smacking for that."

Mel intervened, her small stature was dwarfed by Nicky's six foot frame. Mel held her arms out and tried to calm the situation.

"Come on Nicky, you know she's a silly cow. You've got your interview tomorrow, don't spoil it, don't wreck your chances of getting out of here."

"But she deserves a good trouncing. You saw what she did."

"Yes but you can get her back in other ways. Anne's on tonight. When she lights up one of her spliffs, we can shop her, she'll get sedated. That'll keep her out of the way for a few hours."

"That's not a bad idea," Nicky replied straightening her long skirt and putting her hands down by her side, "Get the bitch one way or the other."

Chapter 7

R noticed a girl sitting in a corner, she was dressed completely in black, the darkness repeated her nail varnish and lipstick. R moved over to sit next to her.

"I don't know you, but you remind me of my son. He's a bit off the wall."

"Thanks."

"Well I just meant that you look a bit different."

"Aren't we all?"

"Right, sorry, didn't mean to be rude but I've been here two weeks and I've never seen you before, are you new?"

"No, I'm long-term, but you spend all your time in the smoker's room and I don't."

"What do you do all day then?"

"Draw cartoons; write poetry, especially when I'm down."

The girl got up and left.

"Who is she?" R asked Kit.

"That's Carla, she's manic depressive but she's getting there."

Although the girl reminded her of her son, he wasn't a Goth, he was just dishevelled. After that on the few occasions when R tried to cut down on her smoking she chatted to Carla about generalities.

"Have you got any brothers or sisters?"

"Yes, nine."

"You must be Catholic," responded R, immediately regretting her lack of tact.

"Well yes, actually we are, do you have a problem with that?"

"Have I put my foot in it again?"

"No, I'm only winding you up. Haven't been to Mass as long as I can remember. Anyway, how many kids have you got?"

"Two, a boy and a girl."

"How old?"

"Peter's twenty and Jo is eighteen."

"Is he fit?"

"Well I think he is good looking, but then I'm his mother so I would say that."

"Is he coming to visit?"

"Not sure because he's at uni and I'm not sure when he can get over."

"What sort of thing is he doing?"

"Creative writing, oh and playing on computer games, writes a bit of poetry, the usual student stuff."

"Sounds interesting, think I'd like to meet him but he seems a bit clever for me. Don't think he'd like my kind of music."

"I think he likes The Smiths, Red Hot Chilli Peppers, he's into lyrics."

"Bet he hasn't heard of Joy Division."

"Seems to ring a bell but he's got so many CDs, I lose track."

One day R saw her leafing through an old photograph album, chewing her top lip as she did

The Women's Ward

so. She fiddled with the loose threads of her thin cotton skirt hardly seeming to take in the images.

"Go on then, what's in the album?"

"Only pictures of my mum and family."

R noticed that her mascara was smudged, there were tracks of black streaking her pale skin.

"So what's the problem?" R asked.

"You know," said Carla, "I always wonder why my mum put me in that home when I was six; there were seven brothers at home. Maybe it was because I was the last one and just too much to put up with. She had me back when I was fifteen when three of my elder brothers had left home."

"Well she must have cared for you to want you back."

"Yes I suppose, but the second time she got rid of me I deserved it. I was on heroin, crack, dope. You name it, I tried it. Don't know why, just did, but at least she bought me a ferry ticket to England and gave me a bit of money. Not much because she suspected what I'd spend it on. Couldn't blame her for that. Had just enough money for my bus fare to Blackpool so had to sleep on a bench that night."

"Weren't you scared? Blackpool gets a bit rough at night."

"Didn't have much option, anyway I had brought the last of my draw with me, so nothing much mattered."

"How did you manage to live?"

"I knew how make money, I'd done it before. You choose a patch, but make sure it's not too crowded, make about two hundred on a good night.

"You don't mean you were a prostitute?"

"Well yes, anyway I'm talking too much, must be in one of my manics. Had to be in their cars. A bit cramped."

"But that was really dangerous; you could have been raped or murdered."

"So you think I don't know? Didn't expect a lecture from you but I was wrong. You're noseying into somebody else's business."

Carla's eyes became small beads of distress. Her nose dripped mucus which dribbled down to the edges of her mouth.

"Sorry," was all R could think to say.

"Don't bother, nobody else does!"

R put her hands to her neck, pressed the bitten fingers into the curve of her throat. Held them there as an act of penitence. She didn't cry because she was trying not to, the nurses recorded any sign of distress and logged it.

"Just fuck off you and go back to the smoker's room, I don't need you."

"Right."

It wasn't, as far as R was concerned.

"Just fucking go."

R began to scratch her arms and take the scabs off the black abrasions she had created with caustic soda, she always picked at them when she got upset.

"So go."

She did.

The Women's Ward

Entering the smokers' room, R observed Denise who was sitting in her usual seat next to the CD player. She had hair like a used Brillo Pad, slightly pink at the edges. Her nose, which was acutely angular, seemed to have been misaligned by a previous accident. As she slept her mouth opened, baby bird-like, waiting for its mother. Her face was scrunched in dreams. R watched the sleeping woman and could almost have liked her for the moment.

Denise woke up before R had taken her first taste of nicotine.

"Right, let me out of this prison!"

She rang the police on her mobile but they already knew her and ignored the call.

"Bastards.   They won't rescue me. Had time when I was out, they were quick enough to arrest me, but now I've been abducted they don't want to know. I will rot here, nobody cares."

After the phone call, her legs began to piston, she banged her high-heeled shoes on the floor.

"Where's my music?"

"On the bloody CD."

"Right you lot, get a life and dance. What's the matter with all of you?" she cried out.

The music was put on at full blast, there was no chance of a private conversation.

"Oh for God's sake, turn it down a bit," shouted Kit.

"Piss off! You just don't know how to enjoy yourself."

Nicky lumbered out of her chair, her larded upper arms dappled with cellulite. She switched the CD off.

"Fat cow, no wonder your husband left you, you are such an ugly cow."

Nicky said nothing, she was used to insults and Denise was a practised bitch.

"Just shut your fat gob or I'll have you."

"Wouldn't dare, or they'll keep you in longer."

The next morning Carla brought her tray over to the table to sit with R who had been bandaged to stop the pus infecting other people's food.

"What have you done to yourself, you silly cow."

"Just an accident."

"Don't give me that."

"You are supposed to be going to a half way house tomorrow. Don't mess it up by trying to help me."

"Well. For God's sake ask for a plaster for that cut!"

R first saw the girl the night she was admitted, being dragged, an assistant on each side holding her under the armpits, her feet slightly above the floor. The ward door was slung open.

R was curious and stopped to see what would become of the new arrival.

"Stop that noise, your fault you feel sick, if you take too many tablets, what do you expect?

The Women's Ward

Now get into that bed, I've better things to do with my time than sit on a plastic chair next to you. I'll send for the duty doctor, he'll calm you down. Sedation is what you need, you stupid girl," the nurse shouted.

"No understand," the girl protested.

"You will soon."

R walked down the corridor in tears. She had turned away, she was in enough problems with the authorities, she was seen as subversive because she questioned, and any intervention was discouraged, but she asked the name of the newcomer from a passing nurse because she wanted to welcome her.

"She's called Elina, but doesn't speak much English, so you lot will have to be patient."

"Aren't we always?"

"In your better times," the nurse laughed," But you do have your off days sometimes."

After two days the girl was allowed out of her room. She appeared to be less than five foot in stature, she wore a short bri-nylon nightdress which had a tear renting its back. The others knew a little of her, being section 4 the door was always left ajar, most patients looked in as they passed. There was little else to do. Other patients were not encouraged to talk to her while she was in her room.

Elina held onto the uprights of the door and stood bare-footed. Someone put out a hand and guided her to a chair, "Here you go poppet."

"What's your name?"

"Elina."

"Here have a cig."

"No do. Me bad, bad person."

"Bollocks, they just make you feel like that. No, you're just upset at the moment."

Nicky put her large forearm around Elina and pulled her gently towards her. Cuddling and stroking her bare arms.

"Just shush, we'll look after you. Come on R, it's drinks time."

"What do you want Elina?"

"No know."

"Look R just bring back a mixture of drinks but don't forget I don't take sugar in my coffee."

Nicky enveloped Elina in her gargantuan bosoms.

Sarah arrived with her clip board to make sure they were mustered.

"You get off her. You know we don't allow physical contact, with your conditions God knows what it might lead to."

"But she was upset; she needed a bit of love."

"No, she's attention seeking. Back to your ward Nicky and come out when you have sorted yourself out," Sarah ordered. "I wish you lot would listen. I know what she needs."

"How come you're only an assistant?" replied Mel.

"Well I've been trained."

"Go on then!"

The Women's Ward

Sarah took a step backwards, shuffled a little before making her reply.

"Well we had a two day induction but it was very intensive. I'm a clinician."

"Bollocks, you're a fucking idiot."

"You know I'll have to take this further, verbal aggression towards staff. Now Elina back to your bedroom, come on, be a good girl."

She went.

The smoke thickened; there was a feeling of impotence which permeated the room. Sarah arrived with her clip board later to make sure none of them had escaped.

R sneaked into her room.

"Come on Elina, don't stay in here by yourself, cheer up, nothing can be that bad and we've got you a drink."

"I need to be punished, wicked, wicked person. Nurse tell me."

"See you haven't learned the rules yet. No night clothes after ten am."

"I no have."

"I'll help you get, I'll let you have one of my dresses," replied Mel.

"God she'll need tent pegs. We'll find her one between us."

"I've got a spare dress but it might be a bit big but I'll try to sort it."

Mel and R only found one dress which might fit Elina's slight frame. Mel had secreted thread and a needle under her cosmetics, sharp things were not allowed. The dress was yellow but she only had white or black cotton. She decided on white but kept the stitching to the back. They sewed it up.

"Here you go, try it on."

Sarah reappeared. She was annoyed that she had been wrenched from her television programmes.

"See they've let you out, but you'd better stop snivelling, or I'll send you back, we have rules here, your country may be different, but we have expectations." Elina crawled into the corner, her dress in her hand.

"Go on, put it on," encouraged Nicky.

Sarah watched the transformation.

"Not bad you almost look British; with a bit of make up you could almost pass."

Elina began to cry again.

"About time you pulled yourself together. You are a real baby."

"Sorry."

"Don't you sorry me, just at least try to be a little bit like a human being, stop wailing and grow up. See, you're still pathetic, I'll write that up in your notes, no home leave for you young lady."

"No," said R, "I just stood on her foot really hard by accident; she'll be alright in a minute."

Sarah went back to the lounge to continue her morning viewing of soaps.

"What a bitch! I wouldn't care but she was only a cleaner a month ago. Who the hell does she think she is?" asked Mel, "Attila the Hun?"

The Women's Ward

"No, you were right, she's just a bitch." R added, "Why do we put up with this?"

"So you think we have a choice. In your dreams."

"But we have the right to be treated with respect."

"And?"

"Well."

"Listen, that's how it is here, naive or what?"

On the fourth day of Elina's incarceration, she was allowed out without an assistant sitting next to her. She was deemed safe or at least less at risk, the targets had been transcribed.

Nicky reappeared with a box of chocolates which she gave to Elina.

"Too kind, you too good."

Chapter 8

Vicky was small, looked vulnerable, her limp reminded Kit of her daughter who had Cerebral Palsy. Kit needed Vicky to be a surrogate daughter because she could only see hers under supervision until she was deemed well enough.

She arrived in the smoker's room in the morning. Standing in the middle, she announced,

"I'm Vicky and I'm a lesbian just in case you wanted to guess."

They didn't; cigarettes were more important.

Kit was more interested in Val's physical difficulties.
"So how did you manage at school, steps and things?"

"Fine, I was just late for a few lessons."

"I'm fighting to get my daughter into a normal school. They say they haven't got the facilities."

"Bollocks"

"Well that's what they said."

"What did they think I needed?"

"Don't know."

"Nothing but my Rosie, she's coming tonight."

Kit had no visitors so awaited the out come through palls of smoke.

The Women's Ward

"Well how did your visit go with Rosie?"

"Well you know how little privacy we get here. At least I'm allowed out for half an hour. We still haven't gone the whole way, thought we could get it on in the quiet room or bathroom but they are opened every fifteen minutes and we wanted longer than that. They had keys to unlock you. They had sliding locks in the main hospital toilet. We were hot for each other."

"What, in a toilet? Yuck! How depraved is that?" Mel asked.

"So you tell me how we could get it on in private when it's pissing down with rain?"

"Doing it in a toilet, that's gross, disgusting!" R added.

"Thought you said you didn't mind I'm a lesbian!"

"What the fuck has that got to do with it? Denise and Zeta both used the hospital toilets. They had excuses, Denise is a whore, Zeta just did as her husband told her. So what's your excuse? It's not exactly romantic, toilets stink, and it's not that you couldn't have left it on hold. What's your problem? You could have waited," argued R.

"Not when you have the hots for each other." Val answered. "Just a week is too long. We needed to touch each other's bodies, the Mile High Club isn't just for heteros. Okay ours was on the ground floor."

"Not funny, it's just degrading using toilets for sex."

"Right, give me an alternative when it's pissing down with rain! You really don't understand, I need her."

"Wish I thought that about my husband," Mel commented, "I can take it or leave it!"

"No, but I'm in love, we need skin-to-skin contact, feel each other's bodies. I put the seat down. Rosy sat on it facing me, I sat and stroked her hair. God, it was a real turn on! She kissed my earlobes, sucking the sleepers, Christ what a turn on! I rubbed her breasts, shame I didn't have any oil, slid my hand down inside her trousers. I was wet for her, but the handle of the cistern stuck into her back so we had to stop."

"Oh spare me the details," commented Mel.

"Fuck off, just because you don't have good sex and I do. It was special, bet you wish your sex life was as good as mine!"

"You're sick."

"No you stupid cow, get real."

"It's not normal."

"Who says?"

"I do, you're strange."

"You know what really puts me off men, they stand up to have a piss and don't even use toilet paper to wipe it, and you have a go at me for trying to get it on in the toilet. Get real."

"But that's natural."

"So I'm not?"

"Well I didn't mean it like that."

"Look don't worry, I don't fancy you, you're not my type and anyway you are far too old for me."

The Women's Ward

R offered cigarettes because she was embarrassed by the arguments.

"Come on, have a fag you lot and calm down. Mary is on duty tonight and you know what that means!"

"Oh shit not her."

Chapter 9

Gwen arrived in the room half an hour before her shift officially started, as she usually did.

"Hello, so what's new?"

The women looked towards her and most of them smiled. It was going to be a better evening.

"You look a bit sad Bab's, you okay?"

She patted her hand.

"What's up my love?"

"John isn't coming to visit for a few days, says he's busy."

"Probably is, tell you what sweetheart, we'll play cards tonight, go in the garden for a bit. Know you don't get out much."

"They won't let me. I tried to get out of the door today, so I'm on ward arrest for two weeks."

"Leave it with me, Sean's on duty tonight, he'll be okay with it."

Gwen bustled to the office, gypsy style skirt swinging.

She returned a few minutes later panting.

"No, you can go out for a sit in the garden with me and they'll even bring our toast and hot drink down. Okay?"

"Sure."

"What's wrong with you R, you've got a face like a month of wet Sundays."

86

The Women's Ward

"Well why can't other staff treat us like real people like you two do?" asked R.

"But you are real people."

"Says who?"

Anne interrupted.

"I was, until yesterday, before breakfast, human or maybe I am God. Why is it a man? Could it be female? I am human at least I was yesterday. I am as confused as a kettle who is never turned on."

"Come on darling, you're just feeling a bit fuzzy today, tell you what, why don't I get you a nice cup of tea and a biscuit?"

Sean arrived and leant on the door surround smiling.

"Just to say drinks will be a bit late because Sue is ill so it's down to me but I expect even I can manage hot drinks and toast."

"Maybe my little muppet, but you are a man so you might struggle," commented Nicky.

"Cheeky effort, I'll make sure you get the soggy toast," laughed Sean.

"Can I see you tonight?" asked R.

"No probs, just give us five minutes. Wait in my office if you like."

She took her Horlicks and toast in but didn't enter; she didn't want to spill anything on his carpet.

He arrived a few minutes later.

R was crying silently, leaning against the wall.

He touched her arm briefly,

"Come on, it can't be that bad, you haven't murdered anyone have you?"

"It's just embarrassing," she sniffed into the tissue he had proffered.

"In you come. I'll unlock the door."

They entered the office.

"Tell you what, you look to the floor and I'll look to the ceiling, will that help?"

"Suppose, but don't know where to start."

"How about at the beginning?" he smiled.

The alarm bell sounded, its red light was insistent.

"Sorry, need to go but wait here for me."

R curled up in the chair holding her problems close. She lost the confidence to explain about Denise, who grabbed their nipples, tried to grab their crotches and always was described as very poorly by the staff. She had lost the moment, even though she knew he would listen.

"Sorry about that. You know how it is."

"Should do. Been here five weeks."

"Come on what's the problem?"

"Oh nothing that's important."

"Look any time, just come back, I'm here. How about after dinner?"

"But you might get busy."

"No, it's a promise."

"Want to talk about Elina."

"Might be difficult. Patient confidentiality etc."

"Don't bother then. Just wanted to know if she is getting better. Won't ask again. Sod you. I thought you actually treated us as human beings but I must have been wrong."

"Sorry but I have to abide by the regulations."

R stood up.

"Sorry, thought you cared. Just forget it."

The next day R felt more cheerful because she had decided to ask her husband to pick her up. If that failed she could use her bank card to take a cab.

"You look happy, what's your secret?"

"I've decided to leave."

"You can't just leave."

"Yes I can, I'm voluntary, not sectioned so I'll go to my review today just to be polite and let them know what I'm going to do."

R waited. She knew she might have to wait maybe until six but it was worth it just to see Dr. King's face when she told him.

It was three o'clock when the nurse came to the door. He looked towards R,

"Right the doctor will see you now," smiled Sean.

He opened the door to the office for her.

"Can you come in with me?"

"Sorry but I'm not your named nurse."

"I think he's called James but he's never even said hello so what does he know?"

"Expect he's read your notes."

"Hearsay, he's no idea."

"Sorry can't comment. In you go then, doesn't look good if you're late. Busy people the psychiatrists."

R walked in.

"Do take a seat."

She chose the one nearest to the psychologist and smiled at him. She was no longer afraid because she was leaving.

"And how are we today?"

"Fine since my detox."

The telephone rang.

"Yes. No, sorry but I'm with a client. Now where were we?"

R noticed that day that his skin was flawless ebony with eyes the colour of sweet chestnuts.

"Fine, really great now. Think I'll go home tomorrow."

Dr. King leaned a little towards her, clasping his hands loosely on his lap.

"Do you think that's quite wise, dear?"

"Yes I'm completely better. No problems at all."

"I know you are improving but you are still quite poorly, I suggest you stay with us for a little bit longer."

The doctor fiddled with his pen and she averted her gaze.

"No I'm well enough to leave. Really I am."

"It's not quite that simple. We had a little meeting this morning and your named nurse and GP feel that you are still at risk."

The Women's Ward

"But the nurse has never even spoken to me. How would he know?"

"See what I mean? You're getting yourself upset."

"But I'm not sectioned, I can go when I like."

"Well no, not at this point in time. Now be a sensible girl, you wouldn't like to force my hand, now would you?"

R gripped the arm of the chair; she managed not to cry but began to shake. She tried to compose herself. Maybe she was far more ill than she believed, and had imagined the conversation.

"C-c- can I go now?"

"Of course. Shouldn't be that long before you get home leave."

There was a knock.

"Come in."

R escaped through the gap made by the open door. She knew she was now imprisoned. Dave didn't call or visit. Maybe, she thought, he was part of the conspiracy for her internment. He was at least good with the dog, taking it for walks and things. He wasn't all bad. Maybe she had driven him to his indifference?

Chapter 10

It was 5.55 two minutes before tea-time. Nicky and Carla stood in the doorway, arms linked. Wiggy was still asking the wall for a scan to decide the sex of her baby, because at sixty-five nothing else would believe she was pregnant.

"Oh for God's sake Wiggy, shut up! Right you two, what happened in Chester?" asked Mel.

"We both got in. It's a great big old house. We're allowed to go out anytime we like and the patients actually run the place, no more locked doors. We go next week," added Carla. "I can't wait. Eighteen months I've been locked up in here. Freedom!"

The bell was rung to indicate that tea was ready. The women filed past the duo into the corridor where the door would be unlocked to allow them into the café. Most hugged or kissed the two as they passed, to celebrate their impending escape. Over tea, Carla and Nicky explained more about their new home.

"You even get your own room, just to yourself. No wards or anything like that, and you're allowed to put posters on the wall."

"Better than that," interrupted Nicky, "you can come and go as you please, apart from meal times. They ask you to be back by ten at night, but I think that's fine though."

"Did you get a meal there?" asked Mel.

The Women's Ward

"You would ask about food. You're a greedy muppet. It was all fresh, no soggy veg and lots to choose from. I might even lose weight."

"It would take a steam roller to flatten all that blubber," laughed R.

"Cheeky bitch. It's all muscle."

"Muscles don't usually flop about."

"Shut your mouth or you don't get back the shoes you lent me."

"Sorry. I was only having a laugh."

"At least I won't have to put up with you when I leave."

Tea was served. None of the women finished their meal. The food was tepid and tasteless.

"Maybe they think seasoning is bad for our mental health; every other thing in this place seems to be!" added Mel.

"Yeah, like we all know Denise is a bitch," Nicky continued.

"Mega cow," remarked Mel.

"No, but she hasn't been outside the ward for a year. Even prisoners get to exercise."

"Oh for God's sake get off your soapbox. If you know so much how come you're still here?"

Nicky placed her hands on the table surface in order to emphasize her point.

"What the fuck is that?" she said. "It's all sticky. Smells like curry."

"Can't be. We had curry two days ago."

"Go then R. Smell it!"

"Shit. I think you might be right."

Nicky scraped her chair back across the brown lino.

"That's it. I'm going to sort those sluts out."

"Calm down Nicky. You don't want to be sectioned again."

"No. I'll be polite but firm."

"You don't do polite!" answered R.

"I'll give it a try for once now I'm going."

"Couldn't I just go and ask for a cloth," R replied.

"No you couldn't. I think I'll show this mess to Alan, maybe he can get things sorted."

Alan followed Nicky to the table.

"Sorry ladies. It looks as if the table hasn't been cleaned for a while. I'll speak to the catering manager about it."

"Well, you wouldn't notice what the café is really like. You're too busy chatting to your friends to see what really goes on."

"Look, I've said I'll sort it."

Having finished talking the women left the table to adjourn to the smokers' room for a while. Nicky went to change out of her Matalan suit and return the shoes she had borrowed from R.

"Right," Mel said, "Now neither of them are here, why don't we have a party for them?"

"Great. I love a party. I've only got 50 pence to last the week, but when my benefit comes in I'll give you a fiver."

The women divvied up and £25 was collected.

"Sorry, you'll have to do the shopping because I'm still not allowed out."

The Women's Ward

"No probs. I'll get a feast with all that money."

"Let's make a list," Nicky suggested. "Right, crisps, nuts, sausage rolls, posh sandwiches, cream cakes and whatever you can think of."

The next week R came back with five carrier bags of fruit juices and food. Alan managed to find some paper plates and some of them cut out doilies from the paper napkins which they were allowed on a Sunday.

They gathered in the lounge and switched Carla's CD player on. Two of them used their sheets to cover the two tables and R put a small flower arrangement in the centre of each.

The patients helped lay out the food, blew up balloons and fixed streamers to the double doors. Even Denise joined in, making a banner with felt-tipped pen and sticking it on the wall with Sellotape. 'Have a good life' it read.

"Right girls, time to get your gladrags on. About ten minutes to lift off. Mel, go and find Carla and Nicky, it's their leaving do tonight," said R.

"The food looks great. What a spread!" said Mel before she left.

R arrived in the room to check the food. The sausage rolls and sandwiches and cakes were arranged on the plates with garnishes and a little side-salad. Sarah entered.

"For God's sake! Health and Safety!"

She disappeared for a few minutes and returned with two black bin bags.

"Have you no idea about possible food poisoning?"

She threw the sausage rolls, sandwiches and cream cakes into the bags.

"You can't eat anything that's not been prepared and cooked in the hospital kitchens. And those flowers will have to go. Someone might eat them."

"Hospital food. Get real! It's usually reheated, congealed, with a skin on it. You have to sieve the stew to find a piece of meat, and then it's a tiny square bit," commented Becky.

"Don't be so ungrateful!" muttered an assistant.

"I'd like to see you try it! You lot send out for takeaways. That says something!" commented Mel.

"Well, we're not allowed to eat with you," Alan replied.

"I see. Being a nutter might be contagious," added R. "You never know, we might infect you with some kind of mental illness."

"No, it's not like that. We have to supervise."

"Bollocks. You all sit there having a chat and never look up unless someone kicks off. You count our teaspoons in and out in case someone uses one as a weapon, but you never notice that Jane always wears a coat in the café so she can put knives and forks in the her pocket."

The Women's Ward

"You should have reported her," Alan said, shifting his weight from one foot to the other.

"You should be watching. Actually, she hides them under her bed."

"Well at least you've told me now. I'll go and check on her ward."

R placed two small wrapped presents on the window-sill. Mary picked them up.

"Right, I'll have to open those. There might be something untoward."

"No, there's a teddy in one for Nicky and a CD for Carla in the other," R remonstrated.

"I'm only doing it for your safety. Rules are rules."

"Oh, for God's sake, Kit spent ages wrapping them up to make them look pretty."

"Don't get stroppy with me young lady or you know what might happen. You think you're leaving next week, but things can change."

Mary ripped off the paper and ribbons. She examined the teddy bear but all she could find was a growl.

"But we've no paper left," R pointed out.

"Well just give them the presents as they are. I don't expect they'll even notice. You could always wrap them up in newspaper."

"I know you search me most times I go out, but this is stupid. Just sod off, you stupid cow."

"That's it. I'm reporting you, you're weekend leave will be cancelled."

R left the lounge. Trying to calm herself she walked several times round the corridors but they were too short to get rid of the bubbling

97

aggression. She had to lean on the peeling paint of the walls to guide her to the threadbare brocaded seat outside the smokers' room.

"Fuck them!" R shouted.

"Come on, you don't normally swear," said Jane.

"Yes, but you don't know what they've just done! Just thrown out most of our food."

R returned to the lounge and sat in the corner sniffing back tears. Mel came in and sat beside her.

"Look we can still give them a send off. I'll get the girls together and let Carla and Nicky know about the party."

The wooden doors clattered as Nicky swept through them. She was resplendent in an ankle length velvet skirt and white silk top. She strode over to R.

"Okay so I've heard what happened but I won't let that silly bitch spoil our fun. I can do crisps and nuts. Now, you miserable muppet, get off your arse and move those tables to the side, at least we can have a dance! I'll get the CD and the others, maybe I can peel Carla out of her pit while she waits for her black nail varnish to dry."

Apart from Wiggy who was still shouting at herself in the corridor, the other women arrived dressed up for the occasion. They partied until one.

The Women's Ward

The next day the usual weekly meeting was postponed until after tea. The women were summoned to the lounge at seven.

"Sorry you had to wait but we had some important visitors today, they needed to interview us," explained Sarah.

"Well, who were they?" asked Carla.

"Don't think you need to know."

"Well I've just said I'd like to know."

"Was it that lot wandering around with clipboards this afternoon?" R interjected.

"It's just part of a survey."

"Well what about?" interrupted Carla.

"Really, you don't need to know. Can't really go into it."

"Why not you silly bitch?"

"No need to be rude Carla."

"Actually I asked the young girl about it. She said it was a survey to see if the government money was well spent, dietary needs, bed space, suicide rates, that kind of thing," added R.

"You don't need to trouble yourselves with that," Sarah the assistant responded.

"Right girls, back to business. Anything you want to bring up?"

"Only my tea," Nicky remarked.

"We don't need that kind of silly comment."

R leaned over to Mel and whispered,

"Don't know why we do this every week. Nothing ever changes."

"Why not say it then?"

"No, I've learned how to behave to get out of here."

"Right, if you two could actually listen we could move on," Sarah snapped.

The meeting dragged on for an hour, R played distractedly with the cord on the front of her veloured chair.

"At least when I go on home leave I might be listened to," she thought. "Maybe he will have missed me, after all, he said he would visit me once, but maybe he was busy."

Chapter 11

At nine-thirty that night Carla rushed into the smokers' room.

"Quick, look what's happening in the corridor!"

R followed her. On a chair next to the office R could see that Denise was sitting astride Elina, her hand up her crotch, the other hand on her left breast. Elina was crying,

"No, please no!"

R ran to the office door but forgot the protocol. She didn't knock because she thought the situation urgent. She tried to explain but was pushed out of the room so forcibly that she hit the opposite wall.

"Can't you read?"

There was a little notice. "Knock and wait for an answer."

"We are monitoring the situation."

She was offered additional sleeping pills to help her calm down.

"Well you won't be needing one because it's you who was in the wrong for ignoring the rules."

"No it's my legal right."

"Don't try and get clever with me, you are in here for a reason."

"Yes and your job is to follow the rules as well, so I'll have the form, please."

"I know what you think you saw but sometimes our mind plays tricks on us."

"Don't give me that, just give me the sodding form."

"No need to be aggressive. I'll need to write that up on your record," the nurse announced.

"I don't give a shit. Just give me the form."

"Well if you insist but I think you might regret it."

This time she had practiced how she would behave.

R had decided to use the skills she had learned at her counselling courses, palms up, passive position, not holding someone else's gaze too long and nodding in agreement. She felt prepared when she was called for and was sure she would win her weekend leave.

She was ushered into the office.

"So how do you think you are doing?"

"Good."

"Unfortunately," he said glancing towards Mary, the assistant. "The other night you totally ignored hospital rules and rushed into office without knocking."

"But it was an emergency. Denise was sitting astride Elina on a chair just outside the office. Denise was massaging her left breast and had her other hand up her crotch. I thought the staff hadn't seen, so I forgot to knock. Carla saw the whole thing. Anyway, that was no reason for Mary to push me so hard that I landed on the opposite side of the corridor."

The Women's Ward

"Now don't exaggerate, she merely reminded you of the rules and guided you outside," added Dr. Rose.

"You're telling lies."

"That's quite enough of that. I won't have my staff's word called into question."

"Well may be it's time you listened to patients."

"You are becoming offensive and aggressive. If you can't be civil I will have to ask you to leave."

"I'm sure you thought you saw Denise attacking Elina but sometimes our minds play tricks on us."

"I may be ill but I'm not delusional. I suppose I imagined Mary saying that they were monitoring the situation."

"Right, I think you had better leave now. Let's hope next week you are feeling a little more rational."

"I expect that means no weekend leave."

"In your present state, I could not sanction it."

"But I know it's my right to fill in a complaints form, so I would like to have the form."

"Well my dear," he said adjusting his tie, "I'll ask staff nurse Sarah to find you one. Now it is really time you left and try to calm yourself. You are clearly very agitated. I'm sure you'll see the incident you think you saw more clearly in the morning. Mary can you go and collect Kit for her review?"

It took until ten o'clock for the form to be found. R wrote about the incident in detail and Carla counter signed it.

She gave the form to a nurse whom she trusted.

"Put it in the internal mail for me please."

"No probs. Somebody rattled your cage?"

"Mary."

"Think it's best for me not to comment."

"Okay but you will post it for me?"

"Yes, said I would so I will."

He smiled and touched her arm.

"Good luck with it anyway."

R returned and spoke to Carla.

"I've done it. Sent in a complaints form."

"Good for you but don't expect a reply. I've written three. No response."

"Well maybe I will because I mentioned solicitors and stuff."

"I haven't got one so I couldn't say that," Carla replied.

"Neither have I, or at least I don't know because my husband deals with that kind of things. But I put it anyway."

"Best of luck."

At eleven o'clock the next day R received a letter with an NHS logo. She rushed to Carla's room to share her excitement.

"Look what I've got."

"What?"

"Look, I think they've replied."

The Women's Ward

R ripped the envelope open while Carla continued to paint her toenails in a shade of aubergine.

"Do you want to hear what they said?"

"Not really but if you want, suppose."

"Here goes then."

'After a full and exhaustive enquiry into your complaint we find no evidence that the staff acted in an inappropriate manner but we are pleased that you felt able to contact us. Please do not hesitate to contact us in future.

Yours R Cowman

Director of communications.'

R wept. Carla looked out the window.

She retuned to the smokers' room in the hope of some consolation.

June was the first to speak.

"Have you ever thought why men don't sit on the toilet when they want a pee? Is it not bendable? Why do they drip-dry and not use toilet paper. They are messy creatures. Just glad I haven't got one."

R did not reply. She looked out of the window and watched the swollen clouds belly up for a storm.

R left the room shaking with anger, frustration and a feeling of helplessness. Her thoughts were a labyrinth of possibilities and she couldn't find the exit. Was she more deranged and confused than she thought she was? Alan, one of the assistants talked to her as if she was normal, but maybe that was part of her therapy, to treat the insane as if they were lucid. The humiliation engulfed her, her hands shook and she began to doubt her own memory.

R leant on the corridor wall to steady herself, things had not gone at all as she had planned, maybe she should have listened to a nurse who had told her that she should remember she was only a client and couldn't put the world to rights. Had Dr. King lied to protect the institution and Mary? She had to stop and hold onto the banister. Carla's room seemed too far away. Once again she was lost.

R tried to focus through her tears. She saw what she thought was a sepia picture of a Victorian asylum. She knew at that point she was a lost cause. The photograph seemed to be a cruel illusion underpinning her lunacy but it was nailed to the corridor wall. Maybe it was a joke or just an oversight by the management.

Nicky picked R up and steered her to their sanctuary.

"Come on you fucking muppet. They'll keep you for ever if you keep throwing wobblies."

R lurched to safety.

She was kept in as being seen as 'fragile.'

"Just behave," the nurse suggested. "You are not the professional here, we are."

She did as she was told and ignored what she believed to be wrong and was pronounced well after the next two weeks.

Chapter 12

Mavis was a favourite with the "clients, always friendly and cheerful. Today she appeared at the door, Hoover in one hand and a bowl of cleaning gear in the other.

"Lovely day, the sun's shining, just the day to get on."

"Do you want us to get out so you can do your cleaning?" asked R.

`"No, it's fine, just lift your feet up when I vacuum."

"Tell you what, wish Mavis could take over the job Sarah pretends to do. At least she doesn't treat us as if we're infectious," Nicky whispered to Mel.

Elina stopped crying for the moment and watched Mavis clean the skirting boards. Mavis stood up slowly and retrieved a cloth from the bowl and some cleaning fluid. Elina picked it up and used the cloth in a circular motion to remove the coffee rings, and emptied the ash trays, and to clean the table legs. Mavis turned,

"You don't have to do that love. But what a brilliant job you've done. You should come and work with me."

"Yes want, me want."

"Go on sweetheart they've rung the bell for breakfast, see you later."

Mavis smiled and touched the girl on the shoulder.

"See you later my love, we'd make a great team."

As the others returned from the canteen they saw Elina through the open door of ward two, she seemed to be smiling, following Mavis, duster in hand. Three days later Sarah saw Elina helping with the cleaning.

"Your job's on the line, Health and Safety, Health and Safety and you young lady, back to your room Elina. You obviously can't be trusted Mavis."

"But she only had a duster."

"You know the rules, abide by them."

Elina was banned from cleaning.

That night she found a needle which had accidentally been left in the back of her borrowed dress. She thrust it into her eyeball in front of the other women.

"Me die, me no good."

"For God's sake get someone."

The nurse ran in after the emergency bell had been rung.

"What's she done now?"

Blood covered her yellow dress but there were no tears this time.

"Stupid bitch, high security for you."

The Women's Ward

Chapter 13

She was let out for weekend leave still medicated, Olanzapined.

"Have you got everything you need for the weekend, toothbrush, your dirty washing, handbag?"

"Oh for god's sake, I've been ill but I'm not stupid."

"Just trying to be helpful, you know how forgetful you are, even when you were normal."

"Yes I've got everything, I think."

Her hesitation was deliberate, to placate him. They got in the car.

"So how has your day been?"

"Denise was horrible to Babs. She called her an ugly, fat cow. Babs cried. The Wig changed her clothes four times this morning. Kit finds most things difficult to remember but Tina has gone home."

"I don't want to hear about the ward."

"Well that's the only place I've been so what am I supposed to talk about?"

"Yourself, how have you been?"

"Good."

They drove in silence. The trees flickered, the snow was granulated.

"Right love, we're home now."

She wanted to say, "I do know what my own home looks like," but didn't. As usual on her weekend leaves she cooked.

"I have to feed myself all week even though I'm working. It's alright for you in hospital you have all your needs catered for."

After dinner he began to read.

"What's that you're reading?"

"A collection of poetry."

"Which poem exactly?"

"Daffodils."

"Uck, I think it's 'chintzy'."

"You can't put twentieth century values on nineteenth century literature. Define 'chintzy'."

"Okay, half-way between twee and tacky."

"'Chintzy' can only be applied to an object."

"Well isn't a poem an object once it's written down. And it's no longer just an idea?"

"Don't be silly."

"Right, I think he is self-consciously being poetic."

"Come on stop trying to be academic, it doesn't suit you. Now can you leave me to get on and you can play with your little story. I'm sure it's therapeutic but with your educational record it won't amount to much, but if it keeps you happy. After all you don't even have a degree, but if it keeps you amused it's a good thing."

He dried her dreams.

"You just go for the sympathy vote. You can't even OD properly, you fuck that up as well, don't die, just cause trouble. I'm just a realist and you're a dreamer. I don't want you to get your hopes up too high. It will just make you more depressed. I am only looking out for you."

The Women's Ward

She didn't reply. There was nothing she could say. She prepared the potatoes and organised the wine and cream sauce for the steak.

R continued to write; her husband having finished The Times crossword, looked over her shoulder and casually glanced at what she was doing.

"Not again, you constantly use the wrong punctuation, how many times do I have to tell you the difference between a colon and a semi-colon?" "I've been reading the Bell Jar," she said hoping to engage his attention.

"That's a bit hard for you, didn't exactly sparkle at you're A-levels, did you? The examiner must have been sympathetic considering your spelling. Let's be honest, academia is out of your sphere."

She couldn't tell him that she had been looking for a word which was so close that she could hear it breathe, the computer seemed to have imprisoned it, and so she collected courgettes and dug potatoes while hoping to of find the elusive word for her 'story'. But she had to make his tea. He liked his meals on time.

"Quite nice, love," he commented after the meal. "Time to go, don't worry I'll do the dishwasher when I get back."

The telephone rang. He rushed to answer it.

"Yes, she's home now but she's not quite well enough to speak to anyone. Yes I'll give her your love."

"Who was that?"

"Jill."

"Why didn't you let me speak to her?"

"Well you're not quite right, are you?"

"Good enough to speak to a friend."

"Being a bit over the top again. You don't want to embarrass yourself. Only trying to be helpful. It's six, need to ring my sister."

Dave did that every night.

"Yes, she's back, been to see one of her fellow alcoholics and of course I had to drive her there. Well alright, as far as it goes, she's not exactly easy to live with. How's mum doing? Oh that bad, but the nurse should have sorted her legs out today. The weather's been quite well here only a bit wet to start with. Yes the kids are fine. Be over to see you next week. Look after yourself."

"Did you have to say, fellow alcoholic, wouldn't a friend have been enough?

"Well who has had to be dried out and spent six weeks in an institution? Not me!"

There didn't seem a point in talking anymore, if there ever had been one. He took her back to the hospital at six thirty. He liked to be prompt.

"See you Tuesday then for your meeting."

"Aren't you coming to visit before then?"

"No point really, you've been with me for three days and I expect they'll let you out soon."

"Right."

He kissed her on the cheek. A nurse pressed the buttons and opened the door.

The Women's Ward

R made her way back to the smokers' room down the short corridor with dark photographs and walls with finger smudges on magnolia paint. She sat down and opened her JPS. Now she felt at home.

"Hi, how did your weekend go?" asked Babs.

"It was okay, well sort of."

"What went wrong? He didn't hit you or anything?" asked Babs.

"No, nothing like that."

"That's alright then. The day they let me out, my Peter gave me a few bruises; mind you I asked for it, not cleaning up and stuff but one of the staff saw the marks so my leave's cancelled and he's not allowed on the ward. I suppose the nurses were looking out for me."

"Silly cow," remarked Nicky. "He'll only do it again."

"But you don't understand, he doesn't do it for nothing, I cause it."

"Bollocks, he's just an evil bastard."

"Mine doesn't hit me, just, well you know puts me down a bit really. Anyway, think they'll let me out on Tuesday after my review."

"Lucky you," commented Babs. "Looks like I'm in here for another two months."

"Well I suppose it will be fine. At least we have a proper appointment time next week. Not hanging around all day."

The trolley trundled past the open doorway, its back wheel squealed against the hard floor, hot drinks would be served soon.

"Right girls," an assistant announced, leaning against the door frame. "Ladies, it's Mary on duty tonight, meds need to be on time."

"Oh God not her. She's evil," Nicky told her.

"No she can't be, otherwise she wouldn't look after people like us."

"What do you mean, people like us? "

"Well, you know."

"You speak for yourself, I'm a damn sight less of a danger to anyone than Mary, compared to her, I'm normal."

A woman arrived in the room, she had square cut false nails and cheap Blackpool jewellery, sixties eye make up, her eyeliner had run a bit and flaked down the left side of her cheek.

"Right you lot, get a move on. Don't forget I expect silence in the queue."

"Who was that?"

"That's her."

"Okay, go and round them all up. You know how stupid most of them are."

The door was open and the conversation with her assistant clearly audible. R backed away from the interaction and returned to the smokers' room but the other women had already left. She caught up with them outside the dispensary. They were stood rigidly against the far corridor wall. Helen was first in line.

"Oh so I see you're on time for once."

"Sorry Mary. Didn't mean to push in."

"No you silly girl, you've got it right, that's a first."

The Women's Ward

The queue moved unusually slowly that night because Helen's needs took time.

"Oh for Christ's sake, hold still, how do you expect me to sort you out if you keep moving? Anyway at your age you should be able to sort yourself out with your own ear drops. I despair of you."

The women shuffled in communal embarrassment for the object of Mary's annoyance. R looked at the notice board again. There was a middle class lady looking benignly from a blue and white poster. PALS, we are here to help you! The noise from the pharmacy interrupted her reading.

"Leave her alone, you know she doesn't understand," R said before she could think better of it.

"You again. I thought you had learned your lesson, when you actually understand about mental health issues, I might listen, just stand in the queue and behave yourself or we might have to change your leaving date."

Mel leaned an arm on R's shoulder and whispered,

"Be quiet, looks like you'll be out in two days anyhow, if you play your cards right."

"Don't know I want to go back."

"Anything is better than here."

R stared at the other posters. She wondered whether she would prefer to be abused or manic depressive.

"Right Nicky, you're next. I thought you'd know better, I expect you in your night attire before meds."

"But I am, I just bought them today."

"They look like something you'd wear on the beach, hardly suitable for sleeping in."

Mary poured the pills into a small plastic cup. The assistant supervised the consumption of the tablets.

"Take her back to her ward, she can stay there until tomorrow. She should know the rules by now."

"Bitch."

"I heard that, some chance of you going to the half-way house. Nasty behaviour I'll write it down in your notes. You'll be in here a lot longer with your attitude."

"Next. Name?"

"Everyone calls me R."

"Well I won't. I presume you have a real name?"

"Well, yes, it's Rita but when I first came in I could only remember the first letter of my name and it sort of stuck."

"Not with me, you are supposed to be in touch with reality by now."

R swallowed her tablets and remembered not to speak again. The pharmacy door was closed, it was time for milky drinks and toast. They wandered to the lounge, lingerie sagging and slippers scuffing the floors. Mel was sat in the corner, her head resting on a table. She was shaking. R wrapped her arms around the other

116

The Women's Ward

woman's shoulders and cuddled her. Mary walked in, she didn't usually fraternise with the patients but this evening was an exception, she was fresh from her holiday.

"Get off her, she's just feeling sorry for herself, she does that often, it's part of her condition. Don't pander to her, you make matters worse. Just go and sit somewhere else," Mary admonished.

R was allowed out for exercise the next morning and bought the cigarettes for the other inmates from the local corner shop.

"Today is probably my last day in here"

"So I suppose we'll have to wait until the paper man arrives in future."

"Expect so."

Dave arrived two minutes before their appointment.

"Worried you wouldn't make it."

"Well you know how it is, lessons to set and things. Hope this is the last time I have to come here for you. Can't keep taking time off you know, just for you."

"You have to say how I did at the weekend. They'll listen. It's down to you really."

"For God's sake, it's you that's ill, not me."

"But..."

"Never mind, it's easy, just pull yourself together and stop being so bloody miserable."

Rita looked out of the window and saw the weather was crying.

"Right Mr and Mrs Carpenter, doctor will see you now."

The two of them followed her, a few feet behind her, down the thin corridor.

"Just try to remember to behave yourself in the meeting," Dave told her.

The door to the interview room was ajar, she could see the huddle of people who made notes in previous meetings but whose function had never been explained. Today she would ask.

"Do take a seat."

Dave sat in the furthest corner on a plastic seat, Rita retained her usual padded chair next to the psychiatrist, she had nearly begun to trust him but she had not quite learned the art of silence.

"My named nurse has told me that I am likely to be released today but before I go, can you explain who those four people behind the oak desk are?"

"Well, students mostly."

"What is mostly?"

"Just staff."

"Maybe you could have explained it to me, I know I was ill but you could have given me a chance to understand, I had enough problems with my own perceptions."

"Glad you are beginning to question things, seems you're on the road to recovery. Look Mr Carpenter, I'll see your wife in six months at out patients. Okay?"

"Yes she needs to be at home. Thanks for your input, you seem to have sorted her out. Thanks again, I'll go and help her pack. "

Her ward was only a few yards away, the carpet studded with chewing gum was the access.

The Women's Ward

"Don't bother to help. Won't be a minute, nearly finished."

She threw the soiled clothes and toiletries into a bag and cried to be going back.

On her return, the dog licked her hand and the little cat busied itself on her lap, at least.

Things went nearly back to the way they were except that she wrote instead of watching afternoon television. On his return from work she was still writing.

"I see you are still messing about again. What's for tea?"

"Potato and courgette bake with sage and apple stuffed pork steaks."

"Oh so you haven't just been indulging yourself?"

"No."

He looked over her shoulder.

"Surely you could just suggest it."

"No, that's how she was, all fucks and muppets, it was part of her character and I won't change it."

"Well if you don't want my help, fail."

He went back to his Sunday Times crossword.

He took her back to hospital at 6pm and was relieved to get rid of her dreams, she, he thought, had no realisation of her limitations.

"How did your weekend leave go," asked Kath.

"It was okay."

Ruth Carter

She dreaded the next time.

Tuesday was review date. He was invited to report back on her progress.

"We've had a meeting with all the agencies and agree that she is well enough to go home with you this afternoon, after the paper work and her medication."

It took two hours to complete the bits and pieces. She packed her case and carried it to the car.

"Well R you're free now."

"So they say."

She kept her dreams of being a writer in her pocket so as not to be judged as delusional. She tried to share just a little bit with some of the others.

"I think I'll write about here. I want to enrol in an inter-active degree course in creative writing."

"Look you need to get a grip. I thought you were better. Do try and be more logical. It's highly unlikely you'd get in, you didn't exactly sparkle at you're A-levels."

"You don't understand, it's an internet course and you don't need qualifications."

"That's a good job then, but don't you think you are over reaching yourself?"

"No."

"Look you will never be an academic you will only get depressed again."

"I've been reading 'War and Peace'."

The Women's Ward

"What made you pick that up? It's too difficult for you."

"I just liked it."

"On a superficial level I suppose. You only got a B for literature. It doesn't say a lot for your understanding. The examiner must have been in sympathetic mode considering your spelling."

"I studied Camus and Dickens."

"But you're not the brightest pebble on the beach."

On the ward, because she was less disturbed than the others, she was considered intelligent; she wanted to go back.

"Just stick to what you are good at, like cooking. A degree is out of your possibilities; don't get your hopes up for something you can never achieve. You don't want to go back there."

"Sometimes... At least the girls didn't put me down."

"It's your silly story, it makes you depressed because you know it's just a pipe dream, you couldn't even be an airport read on your best day. Don't be ridiculous; just stick to what you know."

She had prepared his favourite meal, gone to the butcher's to buy a duck and the grocery store for blackberries for the sauce.

"That was quite good love."

She stacked the dishwasher, went to the attic and took out a suitcase.